MEMORY MANIA

By Kim Evans

Kim Evans

Published by
Chipmunkapublishing
PO Box 6872
Brentwood
Essex CM13 1ZT
United Kingdom

http://www.chipmunkapublishing.com

Edited by Folake Akinbode

Acknowledgements

These memories were written in response to a conversation I had with Michelle Phillips, a saxophone player in the Nottingham Symphonic Wind Orchestra. After a long evening of recounting my story to her she suggested that I write it down.

I would like to thank all the people who have read early drafts of these 'Memories of Mania' and offered me comments about how to make them more accessible to a general public who don't know me. My housemates, Lawrence Taylor and Tim Hetherington were very helpful, as were a number of my friends including James Jobanputra, Nadja van Ginneken and Simon Tcherniak. My parents also offered useful comments on the writing.

There are many people I've met along the way who've helped the story of my mental health issues evolve in its own particular way. My thanks extend to them as well.

Kim Evans

Setting the Scene

My twenties were a fascinating and illuminating decade for me. It was a time of tremendous spiritual growth and change. But as the title of this book suggests, this transformation was set against a backdrop of mental illness. The mania I refer to is the upswing of manic depression (or bipolar disorder); a euphoric and extremely energetic state in which people often report intense feelings of connectedness to everything around them in the universe. In my case, I also experienced delusions of grandeur and an inability to communicate effectively with my friends and other people around me. However, my overall feeling about my experiences, despite their disruptiveness to my life in general, is that the net result is extremely positive. I feel enriched by my life journey; I have had many fascinating encounters and experiences during my manic episodes and feel very strongly that my mental illness has added colour and vividness to my memories.

In my first draft of my memories of mania I attempted to begin the story with my first visit to psychiatric hospital in Edinburgh in June 1995. While this was the first definitive proof that something was amiss, starting the story here left a lot of questions unanswered and it meant that the story was only really accessible to people who already knew me. In order to explain what lay behind my being admitted to the Royal Edinburgh

Hospital it is necessary that I push the start of the story back a bit further.

I had deliberately selected a set of A-level subjects that opened as many doors as possible. (I studied maths, further maths, physics, chemistry, French and general studies.) It is not at all obvious what the next step is for someone who obtains six "A"s in such a set of subjects - there are a phenomenal number of options available. During my sixth form I had been to an open day at Queens' College, Cambridge and had fallen in love with the magical mystique of that ancient university. Maths was the subject at which I most excelled and I was offered a place at Queens' College to study mathematics.

However, during a gap year in India before starting at university I had begun to feel that studying only maths was too limiting; after revelling in the diversity of my A-level years I was loath to confine myself to just one subject. Genetics seemed broader – I read and loved Richard Dawkins' book 'The Selfish Gene' during my time in Calcutta - and the natural science tripos (the Cambridge word for course) appeared to offer plenty of interesting choices. When I got back from India I asked Cambridge about the possibility of changing from maths to natural sciences and after another interview my request was granted.

In the summer holiday of 1993, immediately before I started the natural science degree at

Queens', I was working on a mobile playscheme in Staffordshire, the county I grew up in. Six of us were employed in two teams of three. Each team had a van of sports and games equipment. Each weekday, each team went out to a different village hall in the county, where we set up for the day and entertained groups of youngsters with various activities. It was a great job - the children were energetic and fun to be with and I got on extremely well with my fellow team members.

I went out with the female member of my team for most of the summer. I was living with my parents at the time, paying no rent, and I was earning about £150 a week which was by far the most I had ever earned. I had access to one of my parents' cars (a battered old two-tone brown Toyota Starlet) and I felt extraordinarily free. The hours were good, the work was enjoyable and we loved spending time with each other. It ended up being a summer of mad socialising; it was the only period of my life during which I regularly went to nightclubs. It was not uncommon for the two of us to go to bed around 3am and wake up at 7am to start work at 8am.

The relationship is special sexually; I had sex for the first time on my 19th birthday in August of that year. We'd been out to see 'South Pacific' in Derby as a birthday treat and we ended the night by sleeping together for the first time. What romance!

However, for both of us the relationship caused problems. My girlfriend left a man in Lancaster in order to go out with me - she was studying at university there. For me the troubles really started after I'd left to go to university. In retrospect I should have ended the relationship before I started at Cambridge. At the end of the summer holiday, my girlfriend went back to Lancaster to continue her studies and I went off to Cambridge. At that point neither of us knew that in five weeks' time we would both be back in Staffordshire, she for her reading week and I having already abandoned my BSc.

But I am getting ahead of myself. The backdrop to the start of my fateful month in Queens' College was a summer of loving and a beautiful, bouncy woman who was the only person in the world who knew me sexually. I'd been working with children in a situation in which a degree of hypomania (the technical term for 'a bit high') is extremely useful - the children seemed to respond well to my general ebullience.

From day one of Freshers' Week I threw myself into socialising with such excessive zeal that it rapidly became utterly unsustainable. I had worked my way through a memory system as a sixteen-year-old and knew about techniques for remembering people's names and faces. By the end of my third day at Queens', I knew the names of ninety people. (I counted them that night as I lay in bed before going to sleep.) It got to the stage where I was so infamous around the college for my bounciness that I would introduce myself to someone and they would say, `Oh, *you're* Kim. I've heard a lot about you.' It was a huge (and ultimately insurmountable) challenge for me to go from the absurdly energetic and bubbly state of Freshers' Week to any sort of 'normal' pattern of going to lectures and studying that most people had settled into after a week or so of term.

I was with a fellow natural scientist in a pub one evening. I acted vaguely surprised when we walked in and found there was nobody that I knew. So I just started talking to more complete strangers, treating the pub as a simple extension of the collegiate environment, on the assumption that somehow the whole world wanted to be part of the crazy socialising I was engaged in. My friend made the perspicacious observation that nothing was big enough for me - I acted as though I wanted to expand my social circle to include the whole world. It seemed I wouldn't be satisfied until I had intimate knowledge of everyone on Earth and could walk into any social situation and immediately know everyone.

With the benefit of a decade of mental illness behind me, it is easy for me to recognise a lot of the signs of hypomania in my experience of Freshers' Week in Cambridge. These included an elevated mood, boundless energy, grandiose thinking and a feeling of connectedness and so on, but also a desperate restlessness, an inability to settle, a flagrant lack of stability.

One of my most lasting impressions of the four weeks I spent at Queens' was a feeling that I wanted to study absolutely everything simultaneously. After leaving the intellectual straitjacket of school, where information and knowledge are conveniently (though artificially) packaged into discrete subjects, my time in Cambridge marked the beginning of my realisation of the true breadth of human academic endeavour.

The theme of my wanting to do everything simultaneously was one that would recur in particular starkness during one of my manic episodes much later by which time I was studying medicine in Edinburgh. That time, when I was admitted to hospital, I was in the mood for challenging the staidness of the psychiatrist who assessed my condition. My dear friend James, whom I'd met on the medicine degree, took me into hospital. As usual in my manic episodes, my inhibitions had completely dissolved and I was doing some peculiar things. On noticing that the psychiatrist seemed to hide behind a facade of formality I decided to try and wake him up to his true spiritual identity. He questioned me in a small office and then left to consult with some of the other staff. There was a box of tissues on the desk and I took the opportunity of being in the room on my own to use the tissues to write the words 'Love is all there is' in big, untidy white letters on the desk. When the psychiatrist returned he was shocked to see the mess I'd made of the room. Later, in the corridor outside, I was taunting the doctor about his tie and goading him to take it off and start dancing ecstatically. He felt as though I was threatening him, and began to wonder whether I had the potential to be violent. James, experienced as he was in dealing with me when high, managed to convince the psychiatrist that I was never violent during my manic episodes, and that I was just playing games with the doctor to test him. A nurse who witnessed the events later said to James that what he saw in me was simply a desire to do and be everything at once. Those words have stuck with me and seem particularly pertinent here as I describe what was going through my mind during my time in Cambridge.

My decision to leave Cambridge four weeks after arriving was fuelled by a number of influences. Coupling these influences with my ultra-ebullience led to an explosive situation that I was in no state to deal with emotionally and to my eventually leaving the hallowed corridors of Queens' College.

I had been sent a reading list for the natural science tripos before the summer holiday. I dutifully worked my way through some of the books on the list, particularly those relating to mathematics. When I arrived at Cambridge I was doing what was called maths B - the hardest of the maths courses for natural scientists. We were given a past paper very early on. The paper had twelve questions on it, of which one had to answer six. As I looked through the paper I realised that I could already answer six of the questions with my further maths knowledge together with the extra stuff I'd read over the summer. My feeling was that this made it a bit of a waste of time to study the maths B course - what could I possibly learn from it? (The fact that there were six questions I couldn't answer didn't seem to occur to me. In my hot-headed, impetuous way, I decided that my maths was so good that the maths for natural scientists wouldn't stretch me sufficiently. That was a bit of a disappointment.)

The next thing that influenced my decision to leave was medicine. I soon got to know a number of medical students. They had boxes of human bones in their rooms and were busy poring over anatomy books within the first few weeks of term. I remember feeling that studying the human body was what I really wanted to do. Although I'd never even thought about studying medicine before that point I suddenly felt a burning desire to study medicine.

This feeling was intensified during a weekend visit to my parents' house just before I left Queens'. I was looking through the Cambridge undergraduate prospectus, trying desperately to clarify what I wanted to do with myself. I looked at the structure of the natural science tripos. It is a system that is designed for progressively greater specialisation and most people choose just one subject in their final year. I decided to make a list of all the final year subjects I was interested in. The list consisted of anatomy, physiology, biochemistry, neuroscience, pathology and psychology (among others). When I turned to the medicine page of the prospectus and realised that those subjects constituted a significant portion of the preclinical phase of a medicine degree my suspicion that I was not doing the right subject was confirmed. I felt very strongly that I should be studying medicine.

My financial situation also played a part in my decision to leave. I felt bad about my parents having to support me through university. We had agreed a monthly allowance that I knew was quite low and I had deliberately selected the cheapest possible accommodation in the college. I hadn't set up an overdraft facility with my bank. Once I'd paid my college fees, bought a gown and a few expensive textbooks, I was almost at the end of my money. I remember having a meal of just a baked potato in the canteen one day; I think it cost me 19p. In the back of my mind I knew that I was running out of money and that was a contributory factor in my stopping my degree so soon after it started.

Finally there was the girl I'd met over the summer holidays, with whom I was nominally still going out when I arrived at Cambridge. I received two letters from her in rapid succession in about the second week of term. In the first, she wrote to say she was sorry but she'd got back together with her boyfriend in Lancaster. A couple of days later I received a letter where the tone had changed completely and she said she wanted to be with me again. This emotional upheaval didn't help at a time when I was certainly not particularly stable. I knew that she would be home in a few weeks' time for her reading week so that was sitting at the back of my mind.

Taken together, these five factors were a sufficiently strong force to push me away from Cambridge. I left and got together with my girlfriend again and tried to decide what to do next.

The most important encounter I had in the four weeks I was in Queens' was with Gemma. She is the only person I have stayed in touch with from my brief stay in Cambridge. I met her at someone's party in Freshers' Week. While everyone else busied themselves with getting as drunk as possible, Gemma, a fellow teetotaller, and I engaged in a conversation that was scintillating and extremely genuine. I was attracted by her kindness and gentleness. She was wonderful company. We'd done virtually identical A-levels and we both played the piano and had devoted considerable effort to the study of karate. It was my first experience of meeting someone whom I felt was a kindred spirit.

But I didn't stay around for very long; my thoughts were elsewhere. One final comment may offer some insight into what else I was going through during that turbulent period. When I arrived in Cambridge after my time in India I think I realised that it was no longer possible for me to be the most academically gifted student in every discipline. (Of course that wasn't really true at school either but since I naively convinced myself that maths, further maths, physics and chemistry were the most difficult subjects of all and I was therefore the best A-level student I could live under the delusion that I was special in some way.) I was suddenly aware of what an extraordinary range of subjects was available at university. Although I was registered for a pretty broad subject (natural sciences), it seemed that lots of other subjects (especially medicine) suddenly appeared even broader. I needed space from my erratic thoughts. So my mother picked me up in our yellow VW transporter van with all my luggage and I returned to living with my parents.

As I was looking for a job after leaving Cambridge, an Encyclopaedia Britannica advert caught my eye. They were looking for sales reps and the advert suggested that they would guarantee an income of £1000 a month for the first three months of the job. During one of my school summer holidays I had done door-to-door canvassing for a double-glazing company. It seemed like a good way to learn about how to communicate effectively. I was attracted to the ideas of selling encyclopaedias for much the same reason. I suppose that the fact that Encyclopaedia Britannica was such a wonderful treasure trove of knowledge also appealed to me - what I really wanted was not to sell encyclopaedias but to read them; it was simply a manifestation of my ongoing insatiable appetite for learning.

Anyway, after six weeks of working more than 60 hours a week and driving about 800 miles a week in a car that I bought from a neighbour of my parents, I was worn out. I felt a little cheated; the £1000 a month came with a harsh condition. It was necessary to have given 36 in-house presentations to qualify for the money. I had done about 38 in-house presentations by the end of the month but then my boss rang up each of the people concerned. If both partners in any of the couples I'd presented to were not present then that presentation didn't count. This took my number of presentations down to about 34 so I didn't qualify for the £1000. My boss gave me £500 for a 'near-miss'. By this stage I was hopelessly in debt; I owed my parents about £2000. It was just after Christmas when I threw in the towel and realised that I was not destined to make a fortune selling encyclopaedias. In fact, I was put off selling for life and have never done another sales job since.

I had submitted an application through UCAS to six universities to study medicine. (In terms of consistency this was a vast improvement on the application I made when I was still at school. In that first application the courses I applied for ranged from maths in Cambridge to International Business and Finance with French in Strathclyde - it was a real mixed bag.) One of the six was Cambridge and I was called for interview in December. I was not accepted, hardly surprisingly. The way I told the story at the time was that by the time I returned to Cambridge I had decided that I didn't want to study there. This was somewhat easier than losing face and admitting that I was disappointed about my failure.

Some time after Christmas I was called down to Southampton University for an interview. They wanted me to write a 500 word essay describing why I wanted to study medicine there. A day or so after receiving the letter, before I'd started on the essay, I received an unconditional offer to study medicine in Edinburgh. As this was my first choice (possibly after Cambridge), I readily accepted and breathed a sigh of relief at not having to write an essay for Southampton.

I wanted to find a way of paying off my debt to my parents so I could go away for the summer.

The job I found to pay off my debt was very enjoyable at first. I worked as a Jungle Bungle attendant at a local hotel. The Jungle Bungle was a brightly coloured indoor children's play area, with ball pools, climbing nets and slides. The children had an hour in the play area, and wore different coloured bibs to indicate which session they were in. At the end of each day I went round the Jungle Bungle to clean it and to throw all the balls that had escaped back into the ball pools. Although I had a great time for the first couple of months, I did tire of the job after a while. However, I stuck at it and had managed to pay off my debt by May.

The summer before I started studying medicine in Edinburgh I worked as a waiter in a beach hotel in

Greece. It was another high-energy summer. Although we worked long hours, we had free use of the water sports facilities during our free time. I learned how to sail and went out windsurfing a couple of times. One of the highlights for me was my involvement with the entertainments programme. Each of the departments (kitchen staff, waiting staff, nannies, water sports instructors etc.) had to contribute to evening entertainments for the guests, all of whom were British. For our turn I wrote a Snow White and the Seven Dwarves sketch. I played the role of Snow White (the narrator). It was a great laugh to get dressed up in drag and tell the story in doggerel verse. Various members of the waiting team came on dressed as dwarves and the story gradually evolved. When I returned home after my summer in Greece I was very thin and probably the fittest I'd ever been; waitering and sailing is a great combination for getting in trim. In years to come, May, the medical student I went out with in Edinburgh, observed that I was often thin when I went high. Certainly I think that at times when my metabolism has been faster I have been more likely to go high than at times when I've been a bit fatter.

So in October 1994 I started a medicine degree in Edinburgh University. I was a first year again and a veteran of Freshers' Weeks. I felt confident, happy and very gregarious.

Having learnt from my time in Cambridge that I wanted to have a go at acting, I soon found the university theatre; the Bedlam Theatre. I got involved with the charmingly surreal Freshers' Play which was called something like 'Daniel and the Golden Sandwich'. Everyone who turned up was given a part. My delusions of grandeur reared their head once more as we waited to hear who had which part. I was pretty certain I would be given the lead part or at least an important part. Was I not great? As it turned out I was cast as a rowdy schoolboy - a pretty minor role. Ach well! It was fun, though intensely time consuming, to be involved with the play. I realised then that attempting to combine acting with medicine would be a challenge, and in retrospect I'm glad that I wasn't really much good at acting - it left time for other things, like music for example.

One of the most negative and least helpful assumptions I carried into the start of my medicine degree was the notion that medics were cliquey. Maybe the problem with my thinking was my considering 'cliqueiness' a bad thing. The fact that first year medics spend a considerable amount of time together and often form friendship groups need not be thought of at all negatively. Anyway, I didn't make any lasting friendships with fellow medics that year. Having said that, there were a couple of people who were at the same anatomy dissection table as me with whom I established a good friendship for a while.

I went into my second Freshers' Week a single man, having broken off my relationship with my girlfriend of the previous summer at New Year after leaving Cambridge. Feeling totally energised after my lovely summer in Greece I was in the mood for a relationship when I got to Edinburgh. I ended up in a relationship that probably wasn't particularly useful for me.

I met the woman I went out with for six weeks at a politics debate in the students' union in Freshers' Week. She was older than me and had a worldly air about her. We fell head over heels into a fairly addictive relationship. We were often awake until 2 or 3 in the morning and we spent so much time together that for the first term of my time at Edinburgh I seemed to have very little time for anyone else. This relationship probably ended up contributing to the biting loneliness that eventually tipped me over the edge into mania. I met her a few years after we stopped going out and asked her why she had ended the relationship. She said that she found that my rapid mood swings were difficult to deal with and she felt that during the time she spent with me she was pushed closer to manic depressive tendencies in herself.

To give you some idea of how absurd a situation we were in considers the following exchange:

We were walking home, hand in hand, one evening in Freshers' Week when I realised that she had a ring on the ring finger of her left hand.

'Why are you wearing a ring on your wedding finger?' I asked.

When she didn't reply I realised something was amiss. 'Are you married?' I asked hesitantly.

'Yes', she said, plainly.

'Oh, so what's going on?'

'Let's sit down', she suggested.

When we were comfortably seated she started to tell me a story that should have caused me to run away immediately.

'I've been married for seven years,' she began, 'we live in a house about six miles outside the city centre. But it isn't working at all and we're in the process of sorting out a divorce.'

I had wondered why she was living so far from the university (she cycled in every day; it must have been good for her fitness). Her behaviour and initial reticence about the relationship began to make some sense. For some reason I wanted to present a front of complete unflappability. So I pretended to take it in my stride and reassured her that it wasn't a problem that she was at the tail end of a marriage. I was still happy to go out with her if she felt like carrying on with our relationship.

Soon after this surreal conversation she stopped living with her husband and moved into university accommodation.

Somehow we went out together for about six weeks. The ending was really bizarre and came out of the blue. We'd had some excellent evenings together and I felt we were starting to get to know each other a bit. I was in my room one evening, preparing to go out to meet her. I was shaving when there came a knock on the door and my girlfriend walked in. She looked over at me shaving and said simply 'I don't want this anymore. Goodbye'. With this she walked out, leaving me staring at my reflection in the mirror in a state of total stupefaction. It seemed a suitable ending to a relationship that should probably never have happened. It was executed in such an abrupt way that I felt absolutely no sense of loss and just got on with my life. I'm glad that I bumped into my Fresher's Week girlfriend a few years later; it made sense of the strangeness surrounding our break up.

As far as the studies were concerned, at least the subject felt right. I loved the intellectual stimulation of studying medical biology and anatomy in the first term. I will never forget my first anatomy dissection class. There were about sixty cadavers on steel tables in a huge room that smelled strongly of formaldehyde. We all traipsed in wearing our brand new white coats and in groups of about six we set about the task of following the instructions in the dissection manual to begin cutting up the body. For me it was a symbolic moment. I'd always been pretty squeamish and the dissections in school biology classes had unsettled me greatly. So I was interested to see whether with a few more years of life experience behind me I would be able to face the dissection classes without fainting. In fact, I was so well prepared mentally for the anatomy that I took to it easily and never felt squeamish at all.

I managed to get a reputation for myself among my fellow medical students. I was one of the few students who ever asked questions in lectures and I was therefore rapidly known to everyone on the course. This put a bit of pressure on me. I still prided myself on my ability to memorise names and faces but the fact that 200 or more people almost instantaneously knew my name felt awkward - it was impossible for me to get to know everyone so fast.

One of the other key features of my first year in Edinburgh was Theatresports, an improvised comedy team who gave shows on Friday nights and ran a workshop on Saturday mornings that anybody could go along to. There was a special show on the Friday of Fresher's Week. One of the games they played was a game called 'Freeze'. The idea of the game is that two people are on stage at a time and they have to improvise a scene. The twist is that if at any time anybody else (including audience members) sees an opportunity to replace one of the players and take the scene in a new direction, they shout 'Freeze!', run onto stage, touch whichever player they wish to replace and take the scene somewhere completely different. I made myself known to another group of people by being the first audience member to shout 'Freeze!' and go on stage. I was wearing a slate-coloured suit at the time; a feature that made me particularly conspicuous.

I loved both the Friday night shows and the Saturday morning workshops. Looking back, I realise that my energy levels were so much higher than other people's that I never really succeeded in establishing any rapport with my fellow actors. I was, quite literally, in a world of my own, a hint of the extreme solipsism that would come in later years. The surrealness of the improvised comedy was what I liked. With plenty of suggestions from the audience, every show was different and seemed to shine with a brilliant, dazzling energy.

I joined a couple of societies. I played saxophone with the university wind band and joined a rock gospel choir called Revelations. It was my association with the latter that led to the events around my first hospitalisation in June 1995.

Edinburgh impressed me from the beginning. It is a powerful and grand city in which one can walk for huge distances. It has plenty of open, green spaces and the skyline is dominated by the imposing presence of Arthur's Seat, a volcanic plug in Holyrood Park to the east of the city.

It felt right to be studying medicine. Finally I'd found the right subject (or rather subjects). Over the course of the first year, in addition to medical biology and anatomy, we studied physiology, biochemisty and sociology/psychology. It was varied and extremely interesting. Unfortunately, my ride was still not smooth and most of my time in Edinburgh was punctuated by visits to psychiatric hospital. Given this account of the two years prior to my initial hospitalisation, the diagnosis of manic-depression (or bipolar disorder) makes more sense. My years after school were characterised by an inability to see things through, my being overwhelmed by the seemingly infinite array of options, excessive gregariousness, delusions of grandeur and extremely high energy levels. It is not surprising that I ended up in hospital. As it happened, religion was part of the initial trigger, and Christianity in particular. This fits in with an idea of Carl Jung's. In his book 'Memories, Dreams and Reflections' he states that he felt that for the majority of his patients their mental distress was caused by a lack of spiritual grounding. It has taken me a long time to build a strong model of my personal spirituality and I think that as a result of taking the time to do some 'soul-searching' I have come to a much more stable and balanced mental state.

The first manic episode: the role of Christianity

I've already mentioned the rock gospel choir I sang with during my first year in Edinburgh. Many of the choir members were Christians and this regular contact with Christianity prompted me to embark on a soul-searching odyssey to find my own answers to the questions they would ask me from time to time about my spirituality.

I remember a little book that I took with me to Edinburgh. It was by Tolstoy. It was really three short books in one volume. They were entitled 'A Confession', 'The Gospels in Brief' and 'what I believe'. I read the trilogy during my first year in Edinburgh and found them useful in beginning the process of establishing my relationship to Jesus. Tolstoy's lucid and essentially secular approach to the gospels appealed to me at the time. When writing the book, Tolstoy did not want to consider any of Christ's miracles and decided to exclude them from his analysis. What emerges is a compelling, if a little cerebral, understanding of what Jesus may have been trying to do with his life. I wasn't yet ready to contemplate miracles and Tolstoy's writing offered my predominantly rational mind a comprehensible introduction to Jesus' life.

At this point it seems relevant to mention a series of conversations I had with a medical friend of mine called Helen at a much later date about my sixth form years. Helen saw quite a lot of me when I was high, and in fact very shortly after starting to get to know her I went high as a result of fancying her intensely and feeling the frustration of recognising that she didn't want to go out with me. She stuck by me through difficult times and often came to see me in hospital in the aftermath of (or sometimes during) my manic episodes. The conversations I had with her were extraordinarily intense as I probed deep into the world of perception and delusion. During the conversations about my time in the sixth form, I built up a very vivid picture of myself emerging from the sixth form like a cannonball shot from a fiery cannon. I was part of a small group of friends in the sixth form. We fancied ourselves as a sort of intellectual elite. Over the course of the two years we spent fraternising, we honed our ability to deliver sarcastic, sardonic comments about the people around us who, to our naive eyes, were inferior specimens and losers. (I exaggerate somewhat; we were not quite as odious as that, but there was an arrogance about my friendship circle at school that may have contributed to my eventually going high, and certainly shaped the atheistic, reductionist world view that I carried with me into my first year in Edinburgh.) In my conversations with Helen, I had images of those years as dark, potent and almost impenetrably dense. The theme of cannonballs returned in various other conversations as I built models of human interactions that involved thinking of people as spheres of different colours banging together like balls on some cosmic pool table.

So, as a first year medical student in Edinburgh, I had a hard-nosed scientific mindset lurking in my subconscious. I had not yet even begun to deconstruct my attitudes and hold my dearly held assumptions up to the light of intelligent, adult scrutiny. I was wildly energetic, even in my darker moods, and attacked life with an intellectual ferocity that I loved.

This provides something of the backdrop to the Friday evening in late May, 1995, when I was invited to a 'Grill a Christian' session by a Danish geography student who lived on my corridor in halls. He was a Christian and it was one of his friends who were leading the session. It was an opportunity for non-Christians to meet Christians and to ask questions about faith and about life in general.

I went along to the meeting with the intention of testing the Christians a bit. I was certain that there was no way that 'they' would convert me to Christianity. I viewed it as an excellent opportunity for an intellectual battle about the existence of God.

There were three other non-Christians and a panel of three Christians, one of whom did most of the talking on the side of the believers. I had so many questions that I ended up doing most of the talking for our group. I approached the meeting with an adversarial attitude; it was as though the battle lines were drawn and the two opposing sides lined up.

I felt that some of the answers the Christian speaker gave to my questions were rather glib. They didn't feel like his answers; rather they were the learned responses that some Christians seem to rely on when faced with difficult questions. Still, it was a lively debate and I thoroughly enjoyed the evening. The meeting ended by my being asked the simple yet highly consequential question 'Who do you think Jesus was?'

It was not a question I'd ever given any thought to. However, I launched into an answer. I don't remember exactly what I said but it was along the lines of Jesus being an excellent politician, a fabulous public speaker and a charismatic man. I also mentioned that I thought he was probably very good-looking which helped him command the attention of the people he spoke to. It was in essence a portrait of a secular but nevertheless impressive man. However, I didn't feel particularly satisfied with my answer. It was this dissatisfaction that fuelled my first adventure into the enigmatic world of Jesus.

The meeting broke up and I went back to my room with a vague sense of unease, a feeling that I had not answered the final (and probably most important) question as well as I would have liked. Fortunately I had some time to rectify the situation.

Every year, some time in May, the students of Edinburgh University are granted a four-day weekend. The Victoria holiday consists of a

Monday and Tuesday and comes as a welcome break when exams are approaching. In my first year in Edinburgh the Victoria holiday weekend was immediately after the 'Grill a Christian' evening. Also, Wednesday was a half day for most students including first year medics. So I effectively had a five day holiday stretching out before me when I left the meeting pondering Jesus' true nature. I vowed to myself that by the end of that five day period I would have found a more satisfactory answer to the mystery of Jesus' true identity.

Early on Saturday morning I went to the main library and took out ten books. Some were historical and/or religious texts about Jesus' life. Others were about quantum physics or relativity. One had the grand title 'God and Space-time'. My pile of books was a fine mixture of theology, religion, history, philosophy and contemporary physics. It is interesting that I genuinely believed that if I read all of those books in a weekend I would have an answer to my conundrum about who Jesus was. I was still a bookish intellectual at the time, and invested the written word with an authority that I have since come to distrust. The realm of experience and internal reflection has become more important to me as I've matured, but at the time I was hungry for other people's ideas about what life was all about.

On arriving back at my halls with my pile of books, I proceeded to read continuously for the next 60 hours. I didn't stop to sleep or eat (although presumably I had the occasional toilet break!) I was so absorbed by the ideas that time felt irrelevant. The only thing I was focused on was the reading. It was a remarkable experience; phenomenally intense. As I read I could feel the ideas coalescing, almost tangible in the air around my head. I could feel my mind broadening and expanding to accommodate the massive influx of new information. My ability to read seemed to improve dramatically. I read faster and faster and eventually reached the point where I could (on some level) take in all the information on a double page with a single glance. I say on some level because I certainly wasn't fully conscious of all the implications and links in what I was reading. However, I had the sensation that my mind was an infinitely deep black box, absorbing the material at lightning speed.

Where did all my reading take me? What conclusions did I come to that weekend?

I think my search began with a couple of history books about the life of Jesus. As well as strengthening my understanding of what we know about Jesus the books led I to my first appreciation that the miracles described in the gospels could genuinely have happened. Before then I sided more with Tolstoy and had not wanted to consider the miraculous nature of Jesus' existence. It was the fact that two historians independently ended their accounts of Jesus' life with a statement to the effect that it was difficult to seriously study Jesus' life without concluding that he was divine that led me to reconsider my beliefs.

Of the other books, the ideas that I remember most vividly from that time concerned Minkowski space-time and world lines. It was a consideration of these ideas that led me to reject the notion of free will. (It was a number of years before I came back to accepting that we do have free will, and it is now a very important part of my world view.)

In a perverse way my renunciation of the idea of free will was a very liberating experience. I suppose the feeling that it was impossible to do anything wrong enabled me to do things that I would previously not have even considered doing. I think I needed the lack of responsibility that came with a belief in total predetermination at that time in my life.

In Minkowskian space-time, time and space are unified with time represented as a fourth dimension. In this way our usual concept of 'object' is expanded. Instead of thinking of objects as three dimensional, we can talk about four-dimensional objects, where a four-dimensional object contains all the information about something *throughout time*. This four dimensional object doesn't move; at every moment in time, we simply observe a different three-dimensional slice of the object; it is impossible for us to see the whole object at once, but it is in some sense 'out there' and unchangeable.

Although the actual means by which I reached my conclusion may be somewhat opaque, the main point is that as a result of my mammoth reading session I decided that we have no free will. This rather strange belief remained with me for a number of months, during which I essentially considered myself a pawn or automaton in some huge system. It gave me a lot of insight into life but I feel that my life is infinitely richer now I have dropped the assumption that we are not free.

After I finished reading the library books I remember reading two other books. The first was the gospels of the New Testament and the second was Terry Pratchett's 'Soul Music.' Both of these books gave me revelatory experiences.

When I was reading the New Testament, I came to the section in which Jesus says something like 'what I have done the least of you will do also'. It was a quote that had appeared in one of the historical books about Jesus, but its impact didn't truly sink in until I read it in its original context. It struck me in a very personal way. From that moment on it was as though God was speaking to me directly. The words on the page were suddenly transformed into messages that were aimed specifically at me. That moment marked the start of my relationship with the Divine. A relationship that has blossomed beautifully over the years, it has become a tremendous source of inspiration and sustenance for me. At times, by responding to what I felt God was instructing me to do, my actions have worried the people around me to the extent that they have felt the need to hospitalise me. Nonetheless, I am extremely glad that I have dared to listen to my sometimes crazy inner voice, (but I'm also glad that I no longer need to go into hospital.)

So after reading continuously for two and a half days, I had come to a deep understanding of the interconnectedness of all things. But where was I on my quest for an answer to Jesus' identity?

Interestingly, it was Terry Pratchett's 'Soul Music' that concludes this section of my development. (Note that by the time I turned to this last book of the weekend I hadn't eaten or slept for a long time and my mind was in a highly abnormal state. The links and associations I was making were pretty bizarre and this is part of the explanation for my unorthodox conclusions.)

I remember very little of the story line of 'Soul Music'. I read it rather too fast to pick up the story. More to the point I was no longer reading in order to understand the story. I was simply on the lookout for more 'messages' from God.

Death is a character that appears in many of Terry Pratchett's books. He is the traditional skeletal figure who carries a scythe. He has electric blue eyes and is an immortal. As I was reading a certain passage about Death I experienced one of the most momentous events of the entire eight-year manic phase of my life.

Although I was just sitting in a chair in my room in halls, I felt electrified and connected to the universe in a way that I have never quite recaptured since. I was reading about Death gazing into infinity and Terry Pratchett jokingly said that infinity has a blue tinge to it. At precisely that moment I experienced an explosion of consciousness. My 'bubble of awareness' suddenly expanded out to infinity and time stopped. It is no exaggeration to say that time stopped - it is the only way of describing what it felt like. The 'here and now' became filled with magic. Every detail seemed to be shouting out to me. I became aware of beautiful patterns in everything around me. I no longer felt I was moving; even when I changed position I was still living in an infinitely protracted now. It was a blissful and ecstatic feeling that lasted until I was given large doses of antipsychotics a few weeks later.

Coming back to the subject of Jesus, it was an easy step (in my now logic-free mind) to link Jesus' comment about everyone doing what he had done with my experience of deep connectedness to conclude that I was some sort of Messiah. That was when the fun really began!

I was in a frame of mind in which I was some sort of messenger of God, nobody had any free will and time had no meaning. It is not surprising that I soon ended up in a psychiatric hospital. However I don't want to jump straight to my hospitalisation. There are some things I remember in the build-up to my incarceration. The experiences I had were my first manic experiences and they were great!

One thing I remember is when a friend came round to my room. We talked for a while and then I felt a desperate urge to try and demonstrate what I meant about world lines and fate. I took a £10 note from my wallet and said something like

'What you can see is simply a three-dimensional cross-section of a four-dimensional object. This note's world line includes all the information about the past, present and future of the note. It will pass through the hands of many people during its existence and the sequence of people who touch this note is completely predetermined. I'm going to show you an experiment. We're going to go outside and I'm going to offer this bank note to everyone I see. The key thing is I have no control over who accepts the note; that is written into the note's destiny.'

My friend didn't really understand my high-energy ramblings about world lines but followed me outside as I leapt up and dashed through the door. I was good to my word and offered the note to everyone I saw. Finally, after offering the note to five or six people, somebody accepted the money. 'You see!' I exclaimed triumphantly, 'I had no control of who took the note, but how could the note ever have been accepted by anyone else. Think how much would have to have been different in the universe for that £10 note to pass through anyone else's hands after mine,' and so on and so on.

I felt really proud of myself for thinking up such a cunning way to demonstrate that we have no free will and that we are all like the £10 note, passing from place to place in a pre-determined way. Of course with hindsight I no longer feel that I proved anything profound with that 'experiment', but at the time it just seemed to fit perfectly with my mindset. (One of the features of my mania was an ability to perceptually twist any experience into something that supported whatever line of philosophical reasoning (or lack thereof) I was pursuing. By filtering out anything that didn't fit in with my current model of the universe I reached a state in which absolutely everything seemed to back up my ideas.)

I continued to think about money, fate and the lack of coincidence in life. (At some point well before my mania emerged I had read 'Memories, Dreams and Reflections', by Carl Jung. It was there that I first encountered the term 'synchronicity'. Jung shared the view (that I still hold), that there is no such thing as coincidence in life and that we attract the 'right' experiences into our life for our particular developmental stage.)

It was in one of my medicine lectures towards the end of the week following my bout of reading when a particularly dramatic example of my mania occurred. It was a lecture on pain by a phenomenally energetic cardiologist. He had a peculiar habit of staring at the ceiling as he spoke. But also, he jumped around, shouted and generally used every dramatic gesture imaginable to put across his message. He would quite frequently stop suddenly and say/shout, 'And you ask me... "Do I need to know this?" ... and I tell you ... the answer ... IS ... YES!!' rising to an almost apoplectic crescendo at the end of each utterance. As I sat in the lecture, enthralled by the performance, I felt the beginnings of a daring and exciting idea. I felt I had an important message for the world and where better to start that with my colleagues. So, at the end of the lecture I dashed down to the front before anyone had a chance to leave and began a rapid monologue about coincidence. I spoke extremely animatedly for a few minutes. At one point I said 'There is no such thing as coincidence. It is no coincidence that you are all sitting where you're sitting, listening to me now.' I took my wallet out of my pocket and emptied the coins onto the table at the front of the lecture theatre. 'It is no coincidence that each of these coins is in my wallet; all of them are on a long journey that will pass through the hands of many people.' I finished my 'act' by borrowing from the lecturer. 'You ask me ...Do I need to know this? ... and I tell you ... the answer ... IS ... YES!!' I punched the air as I finished and returned to my seat to collect my bag. After a few moments of stunned silence the assembled medics started to leaved the lecture theatre, muttering among themselves about the madman in their midst.

My parents happened to be in Edinburgh to see me that weekend (a week after I went to the 'Grill a Christian' session). On talking to them afterwards it emerged that they were quite worried about me, which is not surprising since I was hyperactive and speaking very fast. I remember going to the botanic gardens with my parents that weekend. It was an extraordinary experience. My colour vision was radically enhanced (another common occurrence in mania), so looking at the gardens in full bloom was a pretty heady experience. Also, as I read the Latin names of the plants I felt a sense of connection with the past; it was as though I was seeing snapshots of the evolution of the Romance languages which gave me some insight into the roots of English.

The main other thing I remember from that weekend was my parents giving me a copy of the Saturday Guardian when they left on Sunday. As I read through the paper it was again as though every article referred to me directly. One article was entitled 'The most famous musician in the world'. I don't know who it was referring to but I took it to mean that there would come a time when I would be the most famous musician of all time. (Delusions of grandeur are a common feature of mania.) As I was reading the newspaper I began to get a sense that the end of the world was nigh. The messages I was interpreting seemed to be pointing to the fact that the world was about to end in a huge explosion. When I asked the question 'When wills this happen?' my eye landed on an article about the final of the rugby world cup that was going to take place in South Africa in a few weeks' time. Immediately the pieces seemed to fit together: I was the Second Coming of Christ and it was my duty to inform the world that the end was near in order that humanity could solve all of the world's problems and unite in a glorious celebration of the finale. It didn't bother me in the slightest that the time available for this dramatic transformation was only a few weeks - I was confident that if God wanted things to happen that way then God would find a way.

The notion that I was Jesus deserves a bit more explanation. However crazy an idea it was, it did have some basis (albeit rather tenuous). Although the name I use is Kim Evans, I was christened Christon Jan Evans. So my 'real name' is a version of Christ. I also looked at other features of my life (admittedly in a fairly biased way). I took my father's birth sign and my mother's first name to give Virgo Marianne. That was clearly symbolically equivalent to the Virgin Mary. My grandfather's name was Joseph and my great grandfather was a carpenter. I was living in room 112 (i.e. 1 (Jesus) and 12 disciples) in halls and my parents' address had the numbers 40 (days and nights), 13(Last Supper) and 7(perfect world number (4) +perfect divine number (3)) in it. I counted up my close friends and found I had exactly 12 close friends (some of whom were not at all impressed at being called my disciples!). I had six As at A-level and played four musical instruments. Surely all this pointed to only one possible explanation - I was Jesus!!

As I'm sure is clear, I was not in a particularly useful frame of mind, considering that my end of first year exams were coming up. However, fortunately, it didn't take long before my friends decided that I needed to be in hospital. The warden of one of the halls of residence was a psychiatrist and he ended up driving me to the Royal Edinburgh Hospital late one evening in early June at the request of some of my friends who were staying in his hall. I was put on ward 1A, the acute admissions ward, under the watchful eye of Professor Blackwood. It was a ward that I would visit many times over the course of the next few years. I got to know the staff fairly well, as well as some of the regular patients.

On my first visit to the hospital I was still in the frame of mine that everything was happening according to some 'Divine Plan'. Every moment was perfect and it was somehow 'right' that I was in hospital at the time. I initially refused to take any medication, totally convinced that I was perfectly well. (I certainly felt better than ever, with phenomenal levels of energy and a seemingly infinite ability to concentrate.) One question I was asked repeatedly was 'Are your thoughts racing?' My answer was always a very honest 'no'. I didn't have thoughts racing through my mind at all. In fact it was as though the interminable chatter of my mind had been utterly silenced and replaced with a profound and meditative calm. There was a fascinating lack of correspondence between my inner and outer states. On the inside I felt totally serene and at peace, whilst my external actions were often outlandish, energetic and bizarre. I would dance around the ward or sing at the top of my voice. On one occasion I climbed on top of a wardrobe in my room and sat squawking like a parrot. I felt like a silent observer of my own madness. It seemed that my crazy actions were a front for keeping me in hospital until the `right moment' for my release. It was a weird experience; I felt quite removed from my own actions - they were nothing to do with me any more. God wanted me to be considered mad, so mad I was.

My mother came to see me in hospital and stayed a few nights in Edinburgh. On the day before she was due to go back down south she managed to convince the hospital staff to let her take me out for a walk. We went to North Berwick and walked together on the golf course, overlooking the sea. When the staff agreed to let me out with my mother I sensed that the time of my leaving the hospital was drawing near. As we walked on the golf course I was alert for signs from God that would let me know that the time had come to leave my mother. We were at the furthest point from the car when I received my signal; a seagull cried and it seemed to be saying 'Run, run!' So run I did, abandoning my mother on North Berwick golf course. I felt energy coursing through me as I sprinted back across the golf course, relishing the freedom that I had patiently awaited for so long.

I had no idea where I was going. I was living truly in the moment, following my inner voice and listening to my intuition. I hitched rides with a number of drivers. I remember the first was a policeman. I felt a frisson of excitement as I climbed into the passenger seat, knowing that I would soon be on a missing person list. I told the policeman that I wanted to get to the A1 and that I was heading for London. London seemed to make sense to me at the time. If I was to play a part in bringing about the end of the world, then London, with its connectedness to the rest of the world seemed a logical place to be. I had visions of speaking on news networks and meeting famous people. London felt like the city where all the action would take place in the run up to the end of the world.

As my journey south progressed I realised that I was not really heading for London and that my parents' house just north of Birmingham was my destination. (At no point did it feel like a conscious decision - that is simply where I was led.)

My journey from Edinburgh to my parents' house 20 miles south of Derby was not easy. I frequently walked significant distances between rides and it took me about 12 hours to complete the 300 mile trip. I got to Nottingham at about 2.00am. A taxi driver kindly gave me a lift across town, even though I had no money, but I was still about 45 minutes' drive from home. By this stage I was barely able to walk and was extremely tired. I remember praying to whatever deity was watching over me for a lift to my parents' house. Very soon after that a car pulled over. I wearily climbed in and said I wanted to go to Derby, not daring to assume that I might be able to get nearer to home than that with just one lift. We set off and I talked a bit about my journey to the two lads in the front of the car. To my surprise, soon after setting off, the driver asked 'Are you Mark Evans' brother?' I told him that Mark was indeed my brother. It turned out that the driver of the car had been out to a night club with my youngest brother a couple of nights earlier and he lived in Barton-under-Needwood - four miles from my home. It was a staggering piece of synchronicity to end an altogether surprising journey. I was dropped off at the door of my parents' house - my prayer had been answered in an immediate and remarkable way. Our back door was open, my mother having intuited that I may head home, so I locked up and sank gratefully into a deep and restful sleep.

I stayed at home for a few days. My mother returned from Edinburgh the next day and for a little while I was happy to relax with my parents. However, all the time I was with them I knew that I was simply biding my time and that soon I would have to continue my 'mission'.

The call came, a couple of nights later. It was about 3.00am and I was lying awake in bed when the thought struck me to disappear into the night. I sneaked downstairs, put on a pair of slightly ill-fitting boots (that would later give me some of the most fabulous blisters I've ever seen) and a raincoat and quietly left the house. Again I didn't know where I was heading - I just followed my instincts.

Instead of taking the obvious route south on the dual carriageway, I started my journey by walking eight miles along a more minor road. I think I got my first lift just as dawn was breaking. Once again I experienced the exhilaration of being free on the road.

I again had the impression that I was heading for London. I got a lift to the M1 and waited for many hours at a service station. Eventually I gave up waiting for a lift and started walking by the side of the motorway. I walked for about seven miles before coming to a sign for Cambridge.

When I saw the sign for Cambridge I felt a strong desire to go there. I was 46 miles from the city with strength of will that burnt inside me with a furious intensity. In the end I got no lift between the M1 and Cambridge and walked continuously for 15 hours, all through the night. Looking back on these experiences I am amazed at what I achieved without food or money. My only sustenance on these journeys was the occasional glass of water, sometimes supplemented with salt and sugar to aid rehydration, that I drank in pubs along the way.

When I arrived in Queens' College I rang my parents to tell them where I was. I had a phone card that enabled me to phone home by typing in a code; my parents paid for the calls. Then I went to visit Gemma. By this stage my feet were in a terrible state but I was still running on adrenaline. Gemma bought me some food and persuaded me to have a bath and to rest for a while. I lay down briefly but was soon up again, charging around the campus like a madman.

Unknown to me, my mother and a GP friend of hers were on the way to Cambridge to pick me up and take me to hospital if necessary. They found me, but just before our meeting another piece of synchronicity occurred.

I was manically running round when I suddenly felt a change come over me. My demeanour changed and I slowed down to a normal pace. I walked round the corner and met my mum and her friend close to the Porter's Lodge at the entrance to the college. I came across as my normal self so after going to say goodbye to Gemma, the three of us went out for a meal in Cambridge before driving back to my parents' home in Staffordshire. For my mother I think this was the first instance of a set of events that led her to believe that intense physical exercise generally had a calming effect on my mood. She was probably right that exercise often helped, but in this particular case I had definitely not come down from the high, even though I had walked for 15 hours.

For the next few days I stayed at home and genuinely felt no desire to leave. My feet were gradually recovering from the hammering I had given them. I relaxed and remained calm, realising that I no longer needed to be quite so hyperactive.

Gemma came to visit a few days later. I remember a conversation we had round our kitchen table, during which my parents were talking about taking me back up to Edinburgh so I could do my exams at the end of June. I looked over to Gemma. Our eyes met and I raised my eyebrows. It later emerged that she knew that if my parents took me to Edinburgh I wouldn't stay there. She even thought about saying something to my parents but elected not to.

The following day my parents drove me back up to Edinburgh. They clearly had no idea of the ecstatic state I was in and genuinely believed that they were taking me there in order that I could sit my first year exams a few weeks later.

As we drove I idly flicked through some radio stations, listening attentively for inspirational messages or rather for confirmations of my own messianic status. One snippet was about the end of a horse race. The winning horse had a name with 'The One' in it. I deemed this highly significant. (Of course I didn't comment on this to my parents; I'd realised that the time had come to be quiet about my inner revelations and to get on with following my path.)

My memories of the other things I heard on that five and a half hour trip are indistinct but I remember succeeding in interpreting almost everything I heard in a way that seemed to herald the imminence of the Second Coming.

When we arrived at my halls in Edinburgh my parents didn't stay long. As soon as they had left I packed my rucksack and set off for London.

My wallet was still in the hospital but I did have a chequebook and my passport. I was thus able to withdraw £50 from my bank before leaving Edinburgh. With my Young Person's rail card this covered the cost of a train ticket to London so I was saved the hassle of hitchhiking down south. When I arrived in London I wandered onto the streets with no sense of purpose and no idea what would happen next. The first person who approached me was intent on getting money from me. I said I had no money on me but said I could get him some money by cashing a cheque. (I didn't realise at this stage that it is not possible to use a cheque to withdraw cash more than once per day.) The man got rather angry when it emerged that I wouldn't be able to give him any money after all, but he soon left in search of more fruitful 'customers'.

At one point I came across a guy playing saxophone on the streets. I listened for a while before asking him if I could have a go. He agreed and I improvised some jazz for a while. I think that was the first time I ever busked. At least one person dropped a coin in the hat while I was playing (not that I cared; I was simply enjoying the moment.)

After leaving the saxophonist I came across a swanky hotel with a piano in its lounge. I went in and asked whether I could play piano for the evening in exchange for a bed for the night. The manager told me that wasn't possible. (Maybe the wild look in my eye unnerved him!)

I decided to ring my parents. They were surprised and worried to hear that I was not in Edinburgh. They asked me to get on a train to Birmingham and then to take a taxi home.

I got to Euston and explained that I had no money. In the end the man at the ticket desk rang my parents and they paid for my train ticket with a credit card. I caught the last train of the day from Euston to Birmingham. From there I caught a cab for the final 20 miles of the journey. Once again I was definitely ready for sleep!

This time my parents realised that I needed to be in hospital. I spent most of that summer in a psychiatric hospital in Burton-on-Trent. It was fairly luxurious, almost like a hotel really. I had a room to myself with an en suite bathroom. I was put in room number 1 which seemed very appropriate to me at the time.

I was given horrible drugs and my memory of that summer is quite hazy. I was given fairly high doses of chlorpromazine and haloperidol. At times my muscles would seize up until I was given an antidote called procyclidine.

Some of my old school friends came to visit me that summer, but often my concentration span was so short that all I really wanted to do was sleep.

The most memorable patient from that period was a young man who had experienced mania that was quite similar to mine. He too had wept for humanity and also thought of himself as a Messiah. He was studying politics in Newcastle University and was a lively conversationalist. His name was Mark, like my brother. When I discovered that his middle name was Richard I got very excited. Richard is my Brother Mark's middle name and my father's first name. The fact that this chap had had experiences very similar to mine and shared both first and middle names with my brother was an example of synchronicity that appealed to me.

First experiences of antipsychotics

When I first went into hospital and was given chlorpromazine (a powerful antipsychotic), I convinced myself that it was possible to not be affected by the drug if I could simply use my mind correctly. When I was given the drug I was absolutely determined not to let it slow me down. I took an extremely adversarial attitude to the drug and tried to deliberately speed up my thinking to counter the effects. I imagined that if it was possible to break down the word 'chlorpromazine' in my mind I would be able to speed up my metabolism and rapidly get the drug out of my system. I'll give you an example of the crazy, crossword/word-puzzle - like nature of my thinking. (While these were not my exact thoughts at the time, it gives you some idea of how I was thinking.)

Chlorpromazine = c = speed of light = photons = 300000 m/s, m features in chlorpromazine, magazine without ga, remove garage ⇨car ⇨ motorbike ⇨Zen (i.e. Zen and the Art of Motorcycle Maintenance) ⇨Buddhism ⇨Nirvana ⇨emptiness, void, clear, sounds like chlor, clear promazine? Clear prom magazine, prom queen rhymes with chlorpromazine, clear promotion, advert, ad ⇨subtract ⇨take away chlorpromazine ⇨clear advert ⇨clarity ⇨mental clarity = result!

I used this sort of word association and pulling words to pieces at various times when I was high. It was as though I felt I could learn something profound about the world, simply by dissecting the words that made up my thoughts. This obsession with words was another recurrent theme of my mental illness. With a bit of life experience behind me I am now able to see beyond words to the meaningful world that lies beneath, but it has taken me a long time. If we imagine someone pointing at the moon, words are like that finger - while they can be used to point at an underlying reality, they are not the reality themselves.

The story continues; enter a mysterious Polish woman

After spending the whole of the summer of 1995 in a psychiatric hospital in Burton-on-Trent I was champing at the bit and desperate to get out into the world again. I'd had to abandon the notion that the world would end with the final of the rugby world cup since that passed with no sign of the Apocalypse. However I didn't stop thinking of myself as Jesus. Somehow the 'End of the World' was part of the Divine Plan; it was essentially a ruse to take me away from Edinburgh for that summer. I tried to encourage people to call me Christon rather than Kim, but it was never an idea that stuck.

I missed my first year exams due to being in hospital and had to sit them for the first time in September. My parents knew some GPs and I was given access to the medical library in Burton hospital to do some revision for my physiology, anatomy and biochemistry exams in September.

My father took me up to Edinburgh for my exam week. We both stayed in halls.

The exams were probably the most difficult exams I had ever sat. All through school I had done extremely well in exams. I'd always been well prepared and I'd never found them a problem. In September 1995 I found myself attempting exams in subjects I hadn't studied seriously for a number of months that I had revised for under the influence of strong antipsychotic drugs. Even when I actually sat the exams I was still quite sedated and my thoughts were very cloudy.

Somehow I managed to pass two of the three papers, only failing biochemistry. I had a viva for the biochemistry and just failed that, too.

It was decided that I should return to Edinburgh for just the summer term of the following year, as a first year again, to resit the biochemistry exam. I was therefore faced with more time out. I'd already taken two years out and I didn't really want still more time away from university but that was my lot. As it happened a very interesting meeting took place in February 1996, five months into my time away from Edinburgh. For the sake of completeness I will describe what happened in the autumn of 1995 before moving on to the momentous encounter.

I managed to get a temporary job on the pharmacy counter of Boots that was supposed to run from October to Christmas. I was employed to help on the health products counter and to hand prescriptions to the pharmacist. It was fun for a couple of weeks but I soon grew tired of the job. In order to keep myself entertained I started playing 'till receipt bingo'. I would look at the date, time and total on each receipt and notice any interesting patterns in the numbers, (e.g. a total of £10.12 at 10.12am.) Sometimes I would even point these oddities out to the customers, who must have wondered about my sanity.

One of my roles was to advise people about the medicines that were available over the counter. We were supposed to refer any difficult cases to the pharmacist or advise people to see a doctor if necessary. It was in this capacity that I did something that led to my being fired about six weeks into the job.

A woman came to the counter one day asking about decongestants. She said she had tried a few but none of them seemed to work. After offering her a few options and listening to her symptoms, which included headaches and dizziness, I somehow arrived at the conclusion that she might have a brain tumour. I shared this information with her (probably in an extremely flippant manner). Given that I was totally unqualified to opine about such things it is not surprising that my outburst was deemed completely inappropriate.

I'm not sure whether I was overheard by my supervisor or whether the woman complained to the manager. Anyway, a few days later I was called into the manager's office. There were two people in the room. They told me about the incident and (generously) offered me the opportunity to work for the remainder of the week before I had to leave my job.

As I look back on that time I get a sense of how stupid I was. I sincerely hope that the woman who came into Boots with a head cold that day was able to shrug off my fatuous remark as the ill-informed and immature ramblings of a disturbed mind.

I felt very strange as I went home that day. I'd never been fired before and I hope that I will never experience it again. I felt a combination of embarrassment and slight nausea. I was worried about having to tell my parents and the impact of what I had done finally hit me. It was not a good time in my life.

However, life went on. I carried on living at home. A strange thing happened at that time; another piece of (rather morbid) synchronicity.

Unbeknown to me, my mother was suffering from headaches and dizziness around that time. She had a brain scan at a local hospital; the doctors were checking whether she had a brain tumour.

I don't know whether the scan was before or after Christmas. My parents decided to take the whole family on a holiday to Portugal at New Year. The reason for the holiday was linked to my mother's scan - either the holiday was a celebration of the fact that the scan was clear or (if the scan was after the New Year), that holiday was potentially our last chance to holiday together for a while. I don't think my brothers and I knew about the brain scan until later. It must have been a great relief for my parents when the results came back and my mother was clear of any tumours. This is the first time I have told this part of my story. I suppose my being fired from Boots is the part of my story that fitted least well with the idea of being the Messiah. I felt that telling someone they might have a brain tumour is not the sort of thing that Jesus would do, so I edited out that part of the narrative whenever I related my story to others.

I've seen a photo of my family while we were in Portugal. I had a thick, dark beard that dragged my face down. I was feeling rather low for the duration of the holiday and my beard seemed to offer me something to hide behind during my period of depression.

During January 1996 I perked up a bit. By February I was ready to start thinking about what I wanted to do with myself until Easter when I would return to Edinburgh to carry on with my studies.

I decided to go away from home and do some voluntary work. After trying a few places I ended up working in a home for disabled people in Essex. It was there that I met a woman who would prove to be a key feature of my 'Jesus story'.

The home was called Lulworth Court. I had arranged to go down for three weeks. I arrived one evening with my rucksack on my back. The first thing I did when I arrived was to go upstairs to my bedroom and drop off my rucksack. When I came downstairs again dinner was being served. I found myself sitting next to a pretty Polish girl who was spending a few weeks in the home as a volunteer. We had both chosen the same meal, a fact that she pointed out to me with a smile.

The way I have told this part of the story in the past, I didn't know the name of this girl on the first evening. It is just about possible that this was genuinely the case - we may have been working in different rooms all evening - but it seems unlikely that this is really how it happened. Her name is an important part of the story.

When I got back to my room later that evening I found a note on my rucksack saying 'SEX GOD' in bold capital letters. I hoped that it was from the girl I'd been sitting with at dinner.

She knocked on my door at about 11pm after she had finished putting the guests to bed. We sat and talked for a while. I soon realised that she was indeed responsible for the note on my rucksack. She told me her name (I'm calling her Maria here). I asked her for her middle name as well, and it turned out that both of her first two names tied very closely to a character that had been close to Jesus. When I heard this I felt astounded ... here was a girl who clearly fancied me whose name was startlingly similar to someone who had been important in Christ's life. All of my Jesus thinking came back in a rush and I decided there and then that I would marry her. (I managed to wait until the summer before proposing to her but as far as I was concerned I felt like suggesting marriage straightaway.)

The three weeks I spent in Lulworth Court that February were filled with joy and laughter. Maria and I saw each other every day, both during the daytime and after work, and we grew very close very quickly. I remember phoning home at one point and telling my mother I was in love. Life seemed rosy. I bought a copy of `Colloquial Polish' on one of my visits to Southend and started to learn her mother tongue. All in all it was a wonderful start to our relationship.

Watching Maria's interactions with the disabled people at the home in Essex gave me a profound insight into her caring nature. There was such tangible warmth in the way she helped people get out of bed, get dressed or eat a meal. Her love for humanity shone through. I suppose the very fact that she had chosen to spend time, on more than one occasion, at a home for disabled people showed that she was a benevolent and loving individual. But even among the company of other such types Maria stood out. My heart went out to her immediately; there was a genuine sense of connection between us. Even in my mania I was not so obtuse that I decide to devote myself to a relationship with someone solely because of their name - there was a lot more to it than that.

When our time in Essex came to an end we parted with the plan that I would go and visit Maria at her parents' house in Poland at Easter. I went home and worked in a BhS warehouse for a few weeks and saved enough money for a trip to Poland at Easter.

When I arrived in Maria's parents' flat in southern Poland I was greeted by smiles and an enthusiastic welcome. Maria lived with her sister and parents in a flat, high up in a skyscraper, among other similar buildings. There was a greyness to the architecture that was uninspiring. Near Maria's block of flats was a small greengrocers. There was a small play park for children nearby, and a church opposite the residential complex.

Inside, the flat was cosy and welcoming. It had three bedrooms - two fairly small ones for the daughters and a larger one for Maria's parents. The main room in the flat was a combined living room and dining room which contained a dark wooden table and chairs at one end and comfortable armchairs and a sofa vaguely focused round a television screen at the other.

Maria's grandmother lived in one of the other blocks of flats on the complex. She saw Maria's family quite often. I met the grandmother on my first visit to Poland and we got on well despite my lack of Polish at the time. (I was not completely without language – I'd spent the four weeks when I'd been living at home trying to get to grips with the complicated grammar of the Polish language. I think the family were pleased with my efforts to speak a bit of their language. Maria's mother and sister did not speak much English but her father knew a reasonable amount.) Maria was very much a people person. She was an outstandingly perceptive woman who used writing for expressing what she experienced. When I met her she was part way through a psychology degree. She had various academic awards on her bedroom wall. She'd been top of her year a few times and regularly published articles and short stories. Academically gifted and a superb linguist, she once told me a story about a Russian lesson she'd had at school. The teacher had set up a sort of competition. Each member of the class was asked to come to the front and read a passage from the Russian book they were studying. The winner would be the person who could read for longest without hesitating or making a mistake. When my fiancee-to-be took her place at the front of the class she read and read; after ten minutes or so the teacher had to ask her to stop. Her flawless performance earned her another prize that day.

The Easter holiday seemed to go past very quickly. I met some of Maria's university friends and we wandered round her city, stopping sometimes to drink coffee in cafes. We went to a show at a theatre with her parents but I didn't understand much of what went on. It was an intoxicating time and we dissolved in each other's love. Everything felt extremely new and exciting. I spent four weeks in Poland that holiday; it was long enough to begin to feel part of the family. Maria's mother did most of the cooking when we ate together. It took her a while to get used to my vegetarianism but by the end she was preparing some creative and interesting dishes. Maria and I had lots of laughs together. There was a fun-loving and young air between us and we loved each other's company. We were so easily amused and our relationship developed beautifully. However, it was soon time for me to go back to Edinburgh to resit the summer term of the first year of my medicine degree.

During the summer term, Maria and I stayed in touch by phone and letters. I started attending a Polish evening class. I felt deeply committed to my relationship with Maria and felt a deep sense of happiness within me. I was only resitting biochemistry, which involved three hours a week of lectures, so I had plenty of time to myself. As well as writing to Mary, I spent a lot of time teaching myself jazz piano. This concentrated period of piano practice has really stood me in good stead in later years.

Maria and I met up again in the summer of 1996. We started our summer holiday by doing another few weeks at Lulworth Court. We then went out to France together where we joined one of my brothers on a campsite. I worked as a barman and Maria worked in the restaurant, picking up some French as she went along. We worked hard but we were very happy together. I had informally proposed to Maria at the beginning of the summer holiday and told her I would formalise the engagement when I visited her in Poland at Christmas.

MEMORIES OF MANIA

The summer I spent with Maria on the campsite near Dijon was marvellous. My brother was there a few weeks before us and he was desperately overworked. He could barely find time for his running (he typically runs about 60 miles a week), and the pent-up frustration manifested with his excema flaring up. He needed somebody to help reduce his workload and cleverly thought of me. I spoke to Christophe, the owner of the campsite, on the telephone before going out. I explained that I wished to be with Maria for the summer and he suggested that we both come out and work on his campsite.

Christophe picked Maria and me up from the train station in Dijon. In the car on the way to the campsite I started chatting to Christophe in French. However, Maria didn't speak French and Christophe's English was excellent so we carried on the conversation in English. It turned out that Christophe, a man only a few years older than me, had inherited the campsite when his father died. He had very extensive wine cellars and the campsite attracted large numbers of English and Dutch tourists.

Maria and I were given an enormous room in the chateau in the middle of the campsite. It had three double beds in it. We often didn't get to bed until very late at night and we had to get up early so we didn't spend much time in the luxurious room. Still, it was a good base and we had plenty of privacy.

Maria picked up some French quite fast, through working with the French staff in the campsite's restaurant. I think she was probably a bit less happy than I was that summer. The chefs in the restaurant were rather difficult to deal with and this problem was exacerbated by the language barrier.

One good thing that came of that summer was a bit of money. Although we were only paid about £90 per week, we had very little to spend our money on and both managed to save most of our salary.

Overall that summer was an interesting but exhausting experience. It was difficult to carve out any quality time together although I do remember going for the occasional cycle ride when we managed to have a day off together.

I got back to Edinburgh in the autumn. Maria was back in Poland I continued with the Polish evening class. I bought a wonderful two-volume Polish dictionary and spent many happy hours crafting letters and poems in Polish for my girlfriend/unofficial fiancee. It was an extremely creative time in my life and I felt a deep sense of contentment.

Maria and I had such fun together. Whether we were taking people in wheelchairs for walks in Southend, working together on the campsite in France or wandering round her home town, we found plenty of opportunities to laugh and our love strengthened with every passing moment. I felt a lightness of spirit when I was with her (or even when I thought about her during our months apart) that was enchanting.

She was a cultured, urbane woman, and we enjoyed going to the theatre or to art galleries together. Maria had an enthusiastic and open approach to life and she welcomed new experiences. She was generous, creative and inspiring.

I spent the Christmas holiday that year with Maria's family in Poland. By that stage my Polish was much better. I'd been studying hard, both on my own and at the evening class and I could almost follow the dinnertime conversations.

Maria organised a very special holiday for us at the beginning of my stay in Poland. We travelled to the Zakopany mountains and stayed in a guest house for a few days. It was a cold winter; the temperature dropped to -30 degrees Centigrade - the coldest weather I've ever experienced. We went for walks in the snow and threw snowballs at each other. We enjoyed the use of the sauna in the guesthouse. It was magical. By Christmas day we were back with Maria's family.

On Christmas day, Maria's grandmother came over to the flat. With Maria's family and me we were six. The main feature of the Christmas meal was carp. Maria's mother brought out a huge, sizzling fish; head, tail and everything else. They knew I was vegetarian but I had agreed to try the fish. Just in case I was unable to eat the carp, Maria's mother had also prepared some cheese and cabbage dumplings (pierogi) for me.

It was as we were eating the main course, when there was a natural lull in the conversation that I decided to put my fear aside and formalise my engagement to Maria. I'd brought a silver engagement ring with me from Edinburgh. It had been in my pocket throughout the meal and I'd kept anxiously checking it was still there. The time had come to see whether Maria would accept it (although having already informally proposed over the summer I felt pretty confident!)

'I have something to say', I announced in Polish.

The family looked at me expectantly.

My heart pounding in my chest, I got down on one knee and launched into the proposal speech I'd rehearsed in my mind so many times.

I talked about how my life had changed through meeting Maria. I mentioned how happy I was to have spent an entire summer with such a special woman. I'm sure I praised her family and said how enjoyable it was to be welcomed into their lives. I talked passionately about the love that was coursing through me. (Though I'm certain I didn't phrase it quite so pompously in Polish!)

I rounded off my little speech by looking Maria straight in the eye and asking her if she would like to live with me 'jako moja zona' (as my wife.) By the time I reached this all-important question there were tears in the eyes of all the women in the room. When Maria whispered 'tak' (yes), her mother gave a little cry. I presented Maria with the ring, which she loved, and gave her a kiss and a hug. Suddenly everyone was talking at once. I hugged Maria's mother, grandmother and sister and shook hands with her father. It was an animated and exhilarating moment. I felt part of the family in a different way. I was now one of them; the ritual of giving a ring and asking their daughter for her hand in marriage brought me immeasurably closer to the family. For all this romance surrounding our becoming engaged, it would only be six months before I broke off the engagement in a fairly callous manner. I fully deserved the complete end to all communications that sprang from my telephoning Maria at the beginning of the summer in 1997, a matter of days before she was due to come over to Edinburgh for the summer holidays, to tell her I didn't want to marry her.

A note on symbolism

One feature of my mania that characterised the majority of my relationships, but particularly my sexual relationships, was a tendency to view people more as symbols than as thinking, feeling human beings. This is illustrated by my fixation on names. As I desperately attempted to coerce the events and people of my life into a messianic framework, I would look at the names of important people in my life and try to work out how I could spin a Jesus-like story out of those names. Having the name Christon was handy. James and Simon are two people who continue to be close friends. These are both names of disciples of Jesus. (I didn't realise at the time, but there was a time during my years in Edinburgh when I could also count an Andrew and a Nathaniel among my close friends, but I've lost touch with both of them now.) I've already mentioned the Virgo Marianne composite of my parents' personal details and the fact that my grandfather was called Joseph. For the sake of anonymity I'm calling the three long-term girlfriends I had in my twenties Maria, May and Mary; the similarity of these substitutes is not accidental. Their real names also tied together in uncanny ways.

There was a terrible cerebralness to my interactions with people. It was as though any message my heart might have had for me was twisted through the vortex of an over-zealous intellect before I would pay it any attention. Rather than feeling genuine emotions and responding naturally to my feelings, I just locked these 'messy' parts of my consciousness away. When the tension had built up to the point where I could no longer contain it, I would go through a set of experiences that would in some contorted way give those emotions expression. Perfectionism, egocentricity (in the form of total disregard for anyone else's feelings) and a desire to push my thoughts as far from any societal norm as possible were some of the things that lay behind my manic episodes.

Although Maria played a strongly symbolic role in my life, she was also far more than that. When I proposed to her I was genuinely contemplating spending the rest of my life with her. For the first time in my life I was considering the implications of lifelong fidelity. I was 21 when I met her in Essex - younger than my parents were when they met and got engaged. But maybe if things had been a little different our relationship could have worked out. Maria's mother had offered to pay for our honeymoon to Kenya. (That was quite surreal. After I proposed we started to dream about where we might go for our honeymoon. For both of us, the idea of a safari in Kenya was the first thing we thought of. I would imagine that such confluence of thinking is quite a rare thing when a couple tries to decide where to go on honeymoon.)

Maria was planning to move to Britain and work as a psychologist after our wedding and we had plans to travel to Venezuela after I finished my medicine degree. We'd booked the church in my parents' village for our wedding in July, 1998, and I'd even designed the invitations. As soon as I'd returned to Britain after proposing to Maria at Christmas I'd asked an old school friend to be best man at our wedding. The details were laid out but in the end I chose differently. (I'm sure that even if my relationship with Maria had worked out my mania would have shown itself again somewhere along the line. Having said that, during the 15 months I was going out with Maria I was free from mania and not taking any medication.)

One reason I have quoted when explaining why I split up with my fiancee was that I felt that basing my decision to marry her on the fact that her name tied in with my Jesus story was not the foundation for a happy marriage. Some part of me felt that only through moving away from that particular scenario could I ever hope to heal. But my thoughts of myself as Jesus did not go away so easily; names continued to play an important part in my story as I desperately tried to fit everything that happened to me into the straitjacket of my messiahship.

Back to Maria; the events leading to our break-up

The time between my proposing to Maria at Christmas, 1996, and ending the relationship with her in June 1997 was a strange and rocky time for me emotionally.

Our relationship worked fine for the first few months. Maria came to visit me in Edinburgh in February and we had a lot of fun together. At the time I was living in a windowless boxroom, sleeping in a single bed. Amazingly, Maria and I had no trouble sleeping together, even in such cramped quarters. I think I snored at the time but even that didn't prevent our having restful nights together.

My friends James, Simon and Nadja were living together that year. I took Maria round to their house for a meal one evening. It was interesting for me to see Maria interacting with new people. She seemed to fit in well and had no problem communicating in English. The only conversation I remember from that evening involved Maria going into some detail about a dream she'd had about butterflies. As someone trained in Jungian psychology she spoke knowledgably and passionately about the symbolism of the dream she'd had; I remember admiring how well she seemed to understand the inner workings of her own mind.

It was when Maria was over in Edinburgh in February 1997 that we were involved in a bizarre conversation in someone's car. I was singing with the musical medics' choir at the time. Maria came to see us sing in a concert and the conversation took place in the car on the way home. Maria and I were sitting in the back and there were two other medics in the front. As medics, I guess they had some idea of what manic depression is about. Nevertheless, I think they were a little surprised by what I was saying. I was basically telling the story of how I had gone high and how I had come to the conclusion that I was Jesus. With Maria sitting right next to me I talked about how she fitted into my manic story. I think the people in the front of the car were rather embarrassed; they simply didn't know how to respond to my indiscrete disclosures. One of them asked Maria how she felt about this. The amazing thing is that she was not at all fazed by these revelations. She didn't seem to mind playing the role I'd assigned her in my story.

As I've already mentioned, Maria was a psychologist and paid attention to her dreams. Once when I was discussing my Jesus status with her she told me that before she had met me she used to have dreams of having sex with Jesus. Interestingly, those dreams stopped when she met me. Of course this was just grist to my mill - further evidence that I was indeed the Second Coming.

I returned to Poland during the Easter holidays in 1997. The dark shadow that would soon loom over our relationship had not yet shown itself. Our relationship was still going swimmingly and it still felt exciting to talk about our future lives together. We had a wonderful day out at the zoo. It was a great opportunity to learn the Polish names for some more interesting animals than the words for pets that I'd become quite familiar with.

The problem started when I got back to Edinburgh for the start of the final term of the second year of the medicine degree. When I got back from being with Maria, the summer holiday suddenly seemed an awfully long way away. I can only assume that the challenge of maintaining a long term relationship was beginning to tell, since within a few weeks of being back in Edinburgh I'd got off with a couple of different women at parties. There was something exciting about meeting a stranger and getting intimate enough with her to kiss and hug in the space of just one evening. (Only one of the two was a stranger, since the first was a chance encounter with the woman I'd briefly gone out with in my first term at Edinburgh, whom I hadn't seen in the years in between.) I didn't feel it was really like me to have these fleeting encounters, especially when I was in a relationship. (I'd not had all that many girlfriends at school but I liked to think of myself as a faithful person.) Maybe as a sort of guilt reaction I decided, very spontaneously, to pay Maria a surprise birthday visit over the Victoria Holiday (the long weekend in May when I'd gone high for the first time a couple of years previously.) I found a fairly cheap flight from Edinburgh to Warsaw via Brussels, with Sabena Airlines, and just turned up at Maria's flat without any warning.

Maria's mother answered the door and took a second or two to register who I was. When she got over her shock she greeted me with a big smile and a hug and called enthusiastically to her husband to come and say hello. Maria wasn't in; I think she may have been teaching English privately somewhere nearby. Anyway, her mother called her and told her that she had a surprise waiting and must come home immediately. Five or ten minutes later, Maria arrived, breathless with excitement. She'd wondered as she walked home if it could be me, but had immediately put the idea from her mind.

It was great to see Maria. I'm very glad I made that trip to Poland. As it happened, it was the last time we saw each other, and although with hindsight I would say I had in some ways already started to extricate myself from the relationship, our last few days together were spontaneous and happy. Ironically, or maybe appropriately, Maria, having no idea that we would see each other again so soon, had stopped taking the pill. She was going to start it again before coming to see me in the summer. So we didn't have sex during that visit (neither of us liked the idea of using condoms). This added a particular poignance to our last long weekend together, although as is so often the case in life, it is only really possible to savour such poignance after the events have finished telling their story.

When I returned to Edinburgh there were about six weeks remaining before the summer holiday. Maria intended to come to Edinburgh for the whole of the summer, and had arranged some work experience with a psychologist in Edinburgh.

At this stage I must introduce a woman I met while studying medicine, since without her I cannot convey the turbulence of the run-up to the end of that summer term. I'm calling her May. I met her when I dropped back a year in medicine. I didn't really start to get to know her until some time in the second year of medicine. When we first met I was attracted to May's wit, energy and worldliness. She struck me as someone who was very comfortable with herself and seemed at home in any social situation. She had a phenomenally fun-loving spirit and laughed freely and warmly. Before coming to university to study medicine she had done a geography degree and some English teaching. It transpired that she had obtained the highest mark in her geography finals of anyone in Scotland in her year. May was a bright spark with amazing people skills and a delightful earthiness. As well as being a wonderful cook she took great pride in her home and succeeded in creating a remarkably stable and welcoming ambience in the places she lived.

As you might expect from someone who had already demonstrated her academic prowess, May had an extremely positive attitude to work and spent long hours in the medical library. She used to like to work in the basement of the library, tucked away in a corner surrounded by learned academic journals. In the end her efforts paid off and she graduated with a distinction from the medicine degree.

One of May's hobbies was ultimate Frisbee. I went along with her a few times. The other players had a similarly zany sense of humour to May; it was definitely the right social milieu for her. I think the creativity required to play ultimate Frisbee was one of the things that appealed to May. She was a very good artist and gardener as well as being an extremely creative conversationalist. When I met her she was sharing a flat with another Frisbee player. The two of them bounced ideas off each other with extraordinary panache, each taking delight in the other's mastery of linguistic gymnastics.

May and I got on extremely well together. We had no end of lively, witty and wide-ranging conversations. May had done a TEFL (Teaching English as a Foreign Language) course before starting medicine, and she'd worked for one of the language schools in Edinburgh, helping foreign students come to terms with the bewildering idiosyncracies of the English language. She had an extraordinary love of words and this shared passion drew us into many conversations about the meanings of words and their etymology. Our conversations didn't really need to have any content - we were both perfectly happy to banter idly with the other about nothing in particular.

May invited me back to her flat for lunch one day during the summer term before Maria was due to come over from Poland for the long summer holiday. Retrospectively it is easy to say that given that I was engaged to Maria at the time, I was acting inappropriately by accepting May's lunch invitation that day. However, at the time I didn't see it like that at all. I didn't feel that there was any possibility that I was being unfaithful to Maria by having lunch with May. Of course, if it had just been one lunch together then nobody would have thought anything of it. As it happened, our lunch times together became a more and more frequent event until we were spending three, four or even five lunch times a week together, often in May's flat but also sitting in a park or going for walks.

My relationship with May grew stronger and stronger. By a peculiar turn of fate, we had chosen identical options during the summer term of the second year of medicine. We had all our classes together and it was almost inevitable that we should grow very close that term. There was one project for which the year of medical students was (arbitrarily) broken up into pairs. To complete the picture of how much time we were spending together, May and I were assigned to work with each other. It involved travelling out to a suburb of Edinburgh to interview a mother of children under five about her experiences of using the health services. It meant that we spent time chatting on the bus together and planning the project together (often at May's flat). We could not help but see a great deal of each other. We studied together, we helped each other on assignments and we had lunch together most days.

The weather in Edinburgh during the summer that May and I met was fantastic. There were plenty of beautifully warm, sunny days and sometimes May and I sat in the park in George Square absorbing the sun and chatting to each other. The following scene shows you that I was thinking in very peculiar ways at this time and it offers some insight into what happened a few months later.

On this particularly weird lunch time, I took a piece of paper from my bag and drew a timeline of the last few years. Then, through very detailed questioning, I encouraged May to pinpoint the times over that period when she had experienced depression. I drew out her responses as a graph, showing how her mood fluctuated across time. My aim in this rather peculiar exercise was to show that May and I were linked in some way that transcended time. I already fancied May at this stage, and somehow felt that if I could show that we had experienced strange moods at similar times over the past few years then somehow that would show that we were 'meant to be together'. Of course, with a bit of forcing on my part I managed to show almost perfect correlation between our moods - whenever May had been depressed I had been high. (This was really fanciful; the match wasn't brilliant but with the partial filter that so dominated my thinking at the time I was able to convince myself that what I was doing made sense.) I think May probably thought I was crazy at that time but it didn't stop us from getting together a short while later.

During the six weeks between my return from Poland for the surprise visit and the time when Maria was due to come to Britain to share her summer holiday with me, my relationship with May reached a feverish intensity. The strain of keeping our relationship Platonic was difficult for both of us. Basically, I had allowed myself to fall in love with May while I was still engaged to Maria.

There came a time a week or so before my Polish fiancee was due to come over to Scotland when things came to a head. May and I had been talking and walking all evening. It was about 1.00am. We had to find a way to resolve the tension associated with both of us knowing that Maria would soon be staying with me. It started to rain so May and I took shelter in a telephone box. She took the chance to voice her concerns. She said something like,

'Kim, we can't carry on like this. You have to choose between Maria and me.'

It was presented in sufficiently stark terms to force me to face up to the situation I had created.

I asked for a few days to think about my decision. When I got home that evening my thoughts were reeling madly, desperately trying to find a clear path through the minefield of conflicting relationships that I'd got me into. After a great deal of agonising the following day, I felt I'd come to the best possible answer. At the time, I believed that May and I would be studying medicine together for the next three or four years. I found it hard to imagine that my feelings for May would diminish in intensity in that time. Maria, on the other hand, was 3000 miles away and wouldn't be living permanently in Britain until after our marriage which we'd booked for the end of July the following summer.

However strange it sounds, I used mind maps to try and help me decide whether to stay in my relationship with Maria or break off the engagement. I took two A3 sheets of paper and a set of felt-tip pens and started drawing big, colourful spider diagrams representing the two significant women in my life. It was a fairly crazy way to even think about making the life-altering decision I eventually made, but I needed to do something and the creativity of the exercise appealed to me even in my confused and unstable state. When I showed my mind maps to one of my flatmates he said that it was like looking at representations of 'wife' and 'lover'. The mind-map about my fiancee gave the impression of dependability and solidity whereas the other picture was an explosion of excitement, colour and fun. In the end I chose fun as a short-term solution, rather than opting for the known situation of staying in the relationship with Maria.

This talk of attempting to use mind maps to rationalise about my decision to break off my engagement to Maria is all well and good, but it masks another factor that was quite dominant at the time. Once I've explained this factor, you will understand why I talked about choosing May as a short-term solution to my quandary.

Towards the end of that summer term, just before Maria was due to come over, May and I were in the student employment service looking at adverts for possible summer jobs. The Royal Highland Show takes place every year. We saw an advert for people to work as bar staff, waiters and kitchen porters at the show. It sounded like fun. But I realised that if Maria came over from Poland it wouldn't be fair for me to spend the first four days of her visit working long days at a job, the main appeal of which was my proximity to another woman I fancied! So in the end, when May took a firm stance with me in the phone box that rainy evening in June 1997, the allure of working with her at the show for four days was an important factor that influenced my final decision to break off my engagement to Maria.

I rang Maria a day or two before she was due to leave Poland and told her I didn't want to marry her. She was stunned, shocked and generally unable to accept the enormity of what I was saying to her. She said she would ring me back in a few minutes. During the time between our short conversations, she rang my father and my brother Sankie in order to ascertain whether I was high or not. Since neither of them felt that there was reason to believe I was manic at the time, Maria had no choice but to assume that I was in my right mind and that our engagement was genuinely over. When she rang me back she very curtly told me that she never wanted to speak to me or lay eyes on me again and then hung up abruptly. Eight years on, she has kept her word, despite the occasional attempt on my part to re-establish contact. It is probably the most acrimonious break-up I will experience in my life. It took me a very long time to forgive myself for what I did. It's one of the moments of my life I have thought most about since.

She wrote a letter to Hamish - one of my flatmates at the time - which Hamish showed me a while later. After I unceremoniously broke off our engagement she became depressed and went into hospital for a while. Her engagement ring was taken from her by her mother along with anything else that could remind her of me. Beyond that, Maria faded from my life almost entirely, my only knowledge of her life coming second hand from Christmas cards that she continued to send my parents for a few years.

It's interesting to point out a few similarities between the two women in my life at that time. Although the similarities may strike you as trivial and contrived, it is important to appreciate that the spectacles through which I viewed the world were somewhat peculiar.

Both Maria and May was the same star sign. I've already mentioned that I took my father's birthsign and my mother's first name as evidence that my parents represented the Virgin Mary (Virgo Marianne). As a sixth former, when I worked in the local paper shop in my parents' village, I collected all 78 issues of the magazine *Zodiac* and it has been a lasting interest of mine to look at patterns in people's behaviour and attempt to link it in with their star signs. Both Maria and May suffered from depression. They were both women who excelled intellectually in their respective disciplines and they had the same initials. Their names were quite similar and my use of Maria and May hints at this.

The summer holiday of 97

There was a recklessness about the way I made the transition from being engaged to Maria to having a sexual relationship with May instead. Sankie, the older of my two brothers, described me at one point as a serial monogamist. He was perfectly justified in that assessment and the seamlessness of my dumping Maria and starting to go out with May was one of the main things he looked at in coming to that conclusion. I suppose in some ways it was inevitable that by attempting to go from one serious relationship straight into another I would cause myself emotional difficulties somewhere along the line. I simply gave myself no space whatsoever to process how I felt about the hasty (and dare I say it rash) decision I had made. For May and me, the transition felt natural; one day we were just about maintaining a Platonic friendship and the next we dropped that constraint and let the relationship develop in its own way. But that only really makes sense if I decided very early on in that summer term that I was not going to marry Maria. I certainly wasn't conscious of already having come to that conclusion, but my actions seem to suggest that by the time May and I started going out I'd already effectively consigned my relationship with Maria to the compost heap.

May played a little trick on me as a kind of test. The day after the fateful telephone conversation with Maria, May said to me,

'How would you feel if I said that I didn't want to go out with you after all?'

I remember lowering my eyes and appearing sad, but it was all an illusion. It was not a real feeling. In the same way that when I had walked to Cambridge and my mother and her GP friend came to collect me from Queens' College I experienced a sudden change in my demeanour that was uncorrelated with what I was really feeling inside, so when May threw this 'test' at me so I witnessed myself responding in a particular way that seemed quite distant from the elation I was feeling inside. Writing like this, I realise that I was almost certainly high at that time. It is not too surprising; there was so much going on for me emotionally and I maintained an outlook of absurd, even maniacal, positivity. For whatever reason, I was determined not to show any emotion that I thought of as negative. It was immature, emotionally unintelligent and generally unhelpful but that's the way I lived at the time.

May and I did work together at the Royal Highland Show. It was at the show that I started an experiment that lasted about three weeks. I have been vegetarian virtually all my life. I saw a chicken being killed in Zambia, where I was born, when I was 18 months old and that put me off meat. Although I remember eating sausages, mince and pork pies when I was eight or nine, I've been completely vegetarian since the age of about ten, when I was taken to a cattle market as part of a school trip. As a vegetarian, one is frequently asked the question 'Why are you a vegetarian?' You continually have to justify your position and it is not until later in life that you realise that the question 'Why do you eat meat?' is a perfectly reasonable rejoinder to the question; why are meat eaters so often exempt from justifying their dietary habits?

Anyway, I started working at the show as a kitchen porter. The food on offer in the restaurant was very high quality and included venison and salmon. Since I felt I could find no coherent moral argument for being vegetarian I decided to see what all the fuss was about. I went on a three week 'meat fest' during which I tried as many forms of meat as I could find. The venison at the show was rather a rich starting point but I enjoyed the salmon. After the show, I tried duck, ostrich, lamb, pork, bacon and chicken. After three weeks I decided once and for all that meat-eating didn't suit me and returned to a vegetarian diet.

At first glance it seems peculiar that I renounced my vegetarianism so readily just after I started going out with May. However, looking back, it is clear to me that this 'meat fest' may well have been my mania rearing its head once more; it was a way of doing something crazy and utterly different to anything I'd done before and a way of asserting to the world that I was not the person I used to be. In some ways it may have represented the beginning of the long period of feeling regretful and guilty about the insanely cavalier way in which I'd ended my engagement to Maria.

Vegetarianism was an integral part of my identity. By attempting to annul that aspect of myself it was as though I was trying to forge a new identity for myself.

Hidden behind my decision to try and eat meat was recognition that the way I had treated Maria when I so abruptly broke off our engagement was pretty nasty. I think I was struggling to come to terms with the impact of what I had done and, as was so often the case during my years of mania, I didn't deal with my emotions particularly well. It has only recently occurred to me that there may have been an emotional element in my attempt at becoming a meat-eater, but I now realise that food and emotions are often tightly linked. I have no idea whether this is really why I chose to eat meat that summer, but it was certainly a very weird thing for me to suddenly do.

After we'd finished working at the Royal Highland Show, May and I did different summer jobs. May had an excellent summer job that she had already done each year for a number of years when I met her. She worked in a summer school north of Edinburgh as the head of the art department. May spent each summer introducing children to the delights of T-shirt printing, candle-making, jewellery making and silk painting. She was well paid for the work and evidently loved it. I went up to see her at some point during the summer and I was impressed with the way she ran her department. She was extremely professional but also light-hearted and funny. She had a fantastic rapport with the children and got impressive results from them. While I was there we inadvertently broke a strict rule of the summer school, namely that visiting partners were not permitted to sleep in the same bed as the person they were visiting. I say 'inadvertently' because we were simply so tired one night that we fell asleep in each other's arms, fully clothed. (We probably would have broken the rule anyway but as it happened it wasn't a conscious decision.)

I found work for a bookmaker in Edinburgh. It was fascinating to see a part of society that I had never had any dealings with before. Many people were completely addicted to gambling and in many ways I found their lives rather sordid, but I enjoyed the experience nevertheless. It was particularly interesting to observe the manager of the shop, a 55 year old man who had worked in the shop all his life. He had a remarkable facility with calculating the return on the bets that were cast. I had to use a calculator to calculate things like the return on a 50 pence bet at odds of 13-5 but Henry could calculate such things in the blink of an eye; it was extremely impressive.

I had plans to go to France in September to work for three weeks on a youth work camp, but in the end that didn't happen. May had plans to go travelling in California, but as things panned out, that plan was also aborted.

I was sleeping at May's flat on the night of Saturday 30th August 1997. I woke earlier than May and for some reason I turned on the television on the Sunday morning. The channels were all covering the death of Princess Diana. I watched fairly dispassionately for a while before returning to May's room.

'Princess Diana has died in a car accident', I said flatly.

'What?' May groaned through the remnants of sleep.

'Princess Diana died this morning in a car accident in France; the television is full of the news', I elaborated.

'Oh dear. That's terrible.'

May dragged herself out of bed and made her way through to the lounge, where she switched on the television and watched for a while, her sleepiness gradually receding. She seemed stunned by the news, and we didn't say much to each other for a while. I was surprised that May was so interested in the story; she had never struck me as someone who was interested in the lives of the royal family. Having said that, I was aware that it was an historic story, and felt I was watching an event that would dominate the news for a fairly long time.

As we sat having breakfast together that Sunday morning, our conversation kept returning to Princess Diana's death. May was gradually coming to terms with the news of the accident and I thought it wouldn't be long before we moved onto something else and left the morbid analysis of the news behind.

However, for May, for reasons that neither of us really understood, the death of Princess Diana served as a catalyst for a period of depression that lasted a number of weeks. In talking about it later, she said that hearing about the death that Sunday morning seemed to shake some foundational aspect of her psyche. It was as though the basis for her own stability was shattered by her learning that such accidents could happen and she felt a lot less trust in the world after that day.

In the end, May's depression and anxiety meant that she was in no fit state to travel round Baja - she felt worried at the prospect of travelling. So just a week or so before she was due to fly off to America, she cancelled her trip.

My long-awaited trip to France was also just round the corner. I'd bought my train ticket and was really looking forward to getting away. But at this juncture I made another decision that would have a profound impact on the course of my life. As May was feeling in a bad way, I decided to stay with her rather than go off to France for three weeks. The consequences of that decision were far-reaching and ultimately contributed to my leaving the medicine degree shortly after the start of the autumn term.

Both May and I had worked all summer, and we needed a holiday. We went to stay with her parents for a few days. We borrowed one of her parents' cars and set off for a short holiday in Scotland. We intended to drive across Scotland to the Isle of Skye. I remember listening to the radio coverage of Diana's funeral as we were driving along. May asked me to pull over, and we sat together in a lay-by, listening to the accounts of the thousands and thousands of people who had gathered along the route of the cortege. I felt no sadness at all as we listened to the radio presenters describing the scenes in London. But May was very moved by the proceedings and started to cry at one point. As I looked over to her crying, I felt that I would be able to understand what she was going through better if I got into the moment more. I don't know how I did it, but somehow I managed to make myself cry too. If we assume that I was a bit hypomanic at this stage it is easier to understand how I was able to generate tears on tap - I have often experienced fairly labile emotions when I've been high. So we sat in the car and cried together. It was a strange moment and I still didn't feel remotely sad.

May and I made it as far as Fort William on that holiday before May felt too ill to continue. So we made our way back across Scotland, making an abortive attempt to have a night in a hostel in the Trossachs on the way back to her parents' house.

I felt a lot of tension inside me at this time. I desperately wanted to have a good holiday and escape from Edinburgh for a while. I should have just done something on my own and left May to try and deal with her depression herself. But I didn't want to abandon her in her time of need.

I'd not been able to get any of the money back for the train ticket I'd bought for my trip to France and I didn't have much spare cash. In the end May and I did manage to get away for a holiday, but it was a disaster.

We were looking in the travel section of a newspaper one day when we saw an advert for cheap flights to Barcelona. The flights were via Birmingham and cost about £160 each. I had enough money to afford the flight but realised that I wouldn't have much left for accommodation in Barcelona. May loved the idea of going to Barcelona for a week and very generously offered to pay for my accommodation if I paid for my flight.

When I think back to my week in Barcelona with May at the end of the summer holiday in 1997, I get conflicting impressions of the place. Part of me thinks back to the staggering and unusual beauty of Gaudi's architecture and the excitement of the big central street - Las Ramblas - with its street artists and endless rows of eateries. Barcelona is a wonderful city. However, my memories of the city are tainted by the fact that during our week there, May and I went through a very difficult time in our relationship, a time of tension and stress that contributed to my going high after I returned to Britain.

When we flew out of Edinburgh May seemed to be in a happy mood. Her depression seemed to have lifted, and we were both excited at the prospect of having some time away together. But after a few days in Barcelona, she started behaving really strangely. Essentially, she decided that she needed some time alone, and we spent the last few days of the week doing our own thing in the city and just meeting up in the evenings. Even when we did meet up, there seemed to be very little joy in our meetings and I suppose if I had had a bit more emotional intelligence I would have labelled my feelings as frustration, confusion and isolation. As it was, I attempted to pretend that I was completely happy with the situation and tried to make the best of the time in Barcelona. We did have a few good times together, such as the day trip we made to Figueres to see the Dali museum, and the day we each sat for a portrait by one of the street artists on Las Rambles, but overall the trip was not good for my mental well-being and when we got on the plane to come home I felt restless and dissatisfied although I wasn't able to face up to the genuine reasons for my ennui.

My parents live fairly close to Birmingham. Since our return journey was taking us back to Edinburgh via Birmingham and we still had a week or so before the start of term, we had originally planned to spend a few days with my parents on the way back. It would have been the first time May met my parents. Having had a difficult holiday together, I think May was not in the right frame of mind to meet my parents. There was an agonising moment in Birmingham airport. I was still going to see my parents, and May couldn't decide whether to join me or continue to Edinburgh. She was standing at the foot of the escalator to the transfer lounge with conflicting emotions passing across her face. She gave a little cry as she finally decided to leave me.

I arrived at my parents' house with lots of emotions rattling around inside me. I continued to suppress them, trying desperately to maintain a facade that everything was fine.

I went on a shopping trip to Birmingham with my parents and bought a copy of the book 'A Course in Miracles'. It is a workbook for achieving Christ-consciousness and tapping into the miraculous nature of the universe. It is set out in 365 daily lessons, intended as a year-long course in personal development.

I was still able to read quite quickly and settled down to read the large, dense book in the week I had available before going back to Edinburgh.

I remember little of what I read. There were passages about the illusory nature of reality and some about the nature of miracles; they are in God's hands - one cannot choose what miracles turn up when. But the section that most held my interest was about 'The Golden Instant'. It referred to the moment in one's life when you saw through the illusion and experienced perfect connection with the Divine. It was something I felt I had had fleeting glimpses of during my manic episodes, but I was keen to experience a more long-term connection with God.

I was reading a part of the book about pain when a plan began to form in my mind. Pain was described as an attachment to the past (or to reality). The book seemed to suggest that when you were in direct communication with God all pain would disappear and you would be truly free.

My youngest brother had done a fire-walk at some point and had felt spiritually enriched by the experience. I was a great believer that anything is possible and that there are no limits to what the mind can achieve.

I decided on a rather unusual route to trying to access 'The Golden Instant'. Since I am a pianist my hands are very precious to me. I decided that some gesture involving potential danger to my hands would be the most meaningful way to demonstrate the submission to God's will that, under my interpretation, was a necessary aspect of feeling the magnificent connection.

In the end I decided to put my hands in boiling water and 'go through the pain barrier' in order to find God on the other side. I filled a kettle, boiled the water and poured it into our kitchen sink. I then made my hands into fists and plunged them into the boiling water.

I probably held my hands in the boiling water for about five or six seconds. It was agonisingly painful and eventually I withdrew my hands, cursing myself for not being able to transcend the pain on this occasion. As a sort of punishment to myself for withdrawing my hands, I didn't put them under cold water. The skin on the backs of my knuckles blistered in a fantastically impressive way. On my left hand I had a liquid-filled blister that extended across my knuckles and part of the way down my little finger. I still have a scar on my left hand from that day of burning. My right hand was less badly affected, probably because the water was shallower on that side of the sink. My right hand also blistered but I have no scarring on that hand.

My parents were extremely shocked when they saw what I had done to myself. They sent me off to the nurse at the village surgery, advising me to say that I accidentally threw boiling water over my hands while I was cooking. The nurse suggested that I put savlon powder on the wounds (the blisters had burst by this time), and to expose them to plenty of fresh air.

I was in a strange, detached state following my self-mutilation. I was completely emotionless. I had the sensation that I couldn't be affected by anything and it was as though I was simply an observer on my life.

My friend James, a fellow medic from Edinburgh, rang me after he heard about my condition. He said later that it was one of the most difficult conversations of his life. The most difficult part of the conversation for him was my refusal to admit that he existed at all!

During this hypomanic phase, I was not labelling the stimuli I was receiving from the world in any normal way. I felt as though I was pure awareness. When I was sitting on the chair by the telephone in my parents' house having a conversation with James that was not how I was experiencing events. Rather, it was as though I was an infinitely deep, dark sphere, absorbing the information the world was throwing at me without the everyday clutter of a mind. So I was in a state where it no longer meant anything for me to identify myself as Kim Evans. If there was an 'I' present at all, it was an 'I' that observed the world from a standpoint of detached, emotionless perfection - a cold and unflappable atom of the collective conscious, stripped of anything that could link it with a personality or with humanity in general. So, for James, if it's any consolation, during my telephone conversation with him, I wasn't granting myself any sort of existence either. I was simply a witness to a particular piece of the wholeness that is Consciousness and he was witness to a different piece. The whole thing was seamless and continuous and it felt meaningless to talk in terms of individual agents.

My thoughts were so detached and distant that I was refusing to admit the existence of anything as mundane as objects. As you can appreciate, my parents were seriously worried about me. In a state such as this there was no telling what I might decide to do with myself.

The time came for the start of term in Edinburgh. My parents quite rightly felt that I was in no state to travel back up to Edinburgh myself and insisted that I stay at home until I'd got 'back to normal'. I was keen to get back to studying and I was prompted by my parents' decision not to let me leave to sort myself out quickly. Although I wasn't completely back to normal by the time I left my parents, I had changed my thought patterns sufficiently to at least be able to give an impression of my usual self.

In the end I only missed the first two days of the first week and I started going to clinical lectures on the Wednesday. My hands had not completely healed and still looked pretty disgusting, with the bluish-green Savlon powder over the wounds on the knuckles.

Abandoning medicine starts a period of relative stability

The start of the third year of the medicine degree was incredibly disconcerting and uncomfortable for me. In medicine it is common for people to take a year out of their medical studies to do an intercalated BSc. In Edinburgh most people who do this do so after their second year. So in the medicine lectures there were the people from my original year who had finished their BSc degrees as well as the people from the year below (the year I'd gone into when I re-sat my summer term of first year) who were going straight into the clinical portion of the course without doing a BSc. There were also a few new faces - people who had done their preclinical medical studies in Cambridge and had opted to come up to Edinburgh for the clinical phase of the course.

I was in a position where my knowledge of anatomy and physiology was rather hazy, never having had the chance to study properly for my first year exams. My knowledge of the second year material was pretty good, but I felt extraordinary unease at being in an academic context in which I was nowhere near the top of the class.

With me nowhere near the top of the class and no intercalated BSc to my name, my ego didn't know where to run. I simply didn't have the necessary maturity and humility to accept my position and make the best of it.

Another thing I should mention at this stage is my squeamishness. For as long as I can remember I have had trouble thinking about needles and medical procedures in general. I remember feeling faint in an assembly at school when one of the teachers was talking about giving blood. It seems my imagination is very vivid on medical themes; even just talking about operations has often been enough to trigger a phobic response in me. Interestingly, as I said, I had no trouble with the dissection classes in first year anatomy. I think I had so much chance to prepare myself for it that when I got there I was fine.

Looking back over the time immediately before my return to Edinburgh for the start of the clinical phase of the degree, I think that I should probably add trepidation to the list of feelings that I was masking by my hypomanic behaviour. I think I was aware that when I got back to Edinburgh I would be in a difficult situation - I knew my anatomy and physiology knowledge were not as complete or detailed as I would have liked, and I knew that I would have to find a way to deal with my squeamishness as well.

May had gone straight on from second year to third year. We were sitting together in a lecture in the Royal Infirmary towards the end of the first week of the course. I think it was about AIDS. Anyway I felt myself beginning to feel squeamish. I couldn't put my head between my knees because of the arrangement of the seats and I was in the middle of a crowded row. I knew that if I didn't do something I would faint and felt that that wasn't what I wanted to do. I had previously discovered that thinking about maths was a good way to avert feelings of squeamishness, so I started doodling mathematical equations in the margins of my notes. (It worked; I didn't faint!)

May noticed that my mind seemed to be elsewhere. On Sunday morning we were lying in bed together and she made a suggestion:

'Kim, how would it feel if you never had to go to any more medicine lectures and could start going to maths lectures instead?'

My eyes lit up at the suggestion. Maths had always been my best subject at school and changing to maths would give me a great escape route from being a middle-ability medical student - a role that didn't sit well with my (super-inflated) ego.

On Monday morning of the second week of term I went to see the admissions tutor for maths. Not only was I accepted onto the maths degree, but, because of my good A-level grades, I was allowed straight into the second year of the course. (In Scotland a lot of people leave school and start university at 17 and most honours degrees are four years long.) On Tuesday morning I started going to maths lectures. I hadn't done any maths for about five years and at that point I relished the thought of some rigorous mathematical study.

For the next year I didn't look back. I found that I hadn't lost my natural aptitude for maths and with an initial few weeks of hard study I was soon up to speed with my fellow mathematicians. It was exhilarating and I did very well in all my exams. I was doing a number of statistics courses along with the maths courses and discovered that I really enjoyed statistics. I have gone on to do a PhD in statistics which shows that statistics would prove a lasting influence on my life.

My first year of maths (i.e. the second year of the BSc course) was an extremely happy year for me. When my housemates Nick and Hamish moved out I moved out of the windowless boxroom into a large room at the front of the flat. Hamish had had a piano in the room and I later replaced it with a piano that May gave me.

I was playing saxophone with the Edinburgh wind band, I was studying a subject that I was good at and enjoyed and I had plenty of interesting friends from my time studying medicine. I was happy and my mental illness seemed to have receded into the background.

The summer at the end of that year was wonderful. I managed to get a bursary from the maths department to study for a project of my own choosing for six weeks. I didn't do much for the rest of the summer; just lazing about really.

I remember a time during that summer. One day May and I arrived at her house to find the door of her flat ajar with evidence that it had been forced open. I think May was glad I was with her as we carefully made our way in, hoping that whoever had forced the door was no longer inside. The flat was in a chaotic state, with papers all over the floor and the furniture all higgledy-piggledy. The television was gone, as were the stereo and CDs. There was not much more of value in the flat so that was all they had taken. May was quite distraught at the thought that someone had been into her flat and stolen things from her. It was the first time anything like that had happened to her.

The policewoman who turned up was brilliant: cool, collected and professional, and she succeeded in calming May down after the shock of having her flat wrecked by some pilferer.

It was this theft that prompted May to start thinking seriously about moving out and buying a place of her own. When her grandmother had died, May had inherited some money. She used this as a deposit on a flat, and moved in soon after the break-in. The place she moved to would come to have many memories for me during the manic episodes that followed. I would often attempt to turn to May when I was high - she really got a pretty rough deal from my mental illness.

After the summer holiday I went into the third year of the maths degree. Having enjoyed the statistics so much, I decided to study for a joint maths and statistics degree. That meant that I had to study a total of eight statistics modules and eight maths modules spread out over the third and fourth years of the course. In my third year I opted for five maths modules and three statistics modules, which meant that in the fourth year I would have to do five statistics modules and only three maths modules.

The first half of that academic year was a delight. I was exuberant, happy and focused on my work, and my relationship with May continued to flourish. I found the modules I'd chosen really interesting and my studies left me plenty of time to read, play music and see friends.

The return to chaos

In 1999, during the Easter holiday of the third year of the maths degree, I went home to visit my parents. Easter was often a time when I went high, as was the summer - probably because I was on holiday from university and had more time to think spiritual thoughts and generally let my alter ego show through. (There is also the fact that Easter is such a central part of the Jesus story.) I continued the theme of experimenting with pain that I had began by plunging my hands into boiling water. I remember going for a walk, barefoot, in the fields around my parents' house. (Having no shoes was to be a recurrent theme that year.) I walked through fields covered in straw, thistles and stones. It was a painful experience but I was indifferent to the pain. I was absolutely determined to learn how to overcome pain and ploughed on. I made no effort to avoid thistles and by the time I finished my walk the skin on the soles of my feet were full of tiny fragments of straw and spines from the thistles.

At one point I came to a river that runs close to my parents' house. As well as attempting to overcome pain, I was in the process of eliminating fear from my life. I decided to swim across the river. The current was strong and there were lots of weeds on the bottom of the river, but I made it across and felt invigorated and alive.

I eventually came out onto the dual carriageway that passes my parents' village and started walking back towards home. By this stage I had taken my top off and was bare-chested. My father happened to be driving past and stopped on seeing me. He was distinctly unimpressed to discover me walking along the dual carriageway, wearing neither shoes nor jumper and was obviously rather worried about me.

On that occasion I was only high for a little while and was well enough by the end of the Easter holiday to return to my maths studies. At the end of the summer term I sat my third year exams. At the time I was registered on a joint maths and statistics degree. I did fairly well in the exams, but felt that my performance was affected by having been into hospital at Easter.

The chaotic summer of 1999

The summer of 1999, after I finished the third year of maths, was one of the most fascinating yet disconcerting periods in my story. My mania took the form of 'rapid cycling' – I was high most of the time and my mood was very unstable. I went into hospital a lot that summer. The only paid work I did that summer was playing jazz piano with a jazz group in a café called café Dix-Neuf. I had far too much free time on my hands and used it to continue my exploration of the boundaries of consciousness.

It was a confusing time and it is challenging to draw out of my memories a clear narrative. This section is therefore presented as a string of wild and confusing manic experiences. This is a true representation of my mental state at the time. I was in and out of hospital many times and the whole summer was wild, exploratory and strange.

I didn't sleep much that summer and many of my most memorable experiences took place at night when everyone else was asleep. I could then really push the boundaries of social acceptability without anyone 'interfering' with my plans and taking me off to hospital.

One of my happiest memories of all time occurred at about 3am on a beautiful, clear night in summer 1999. At the time I was living close to Arthur's Seat - a hill that commands a fabulous view out over Edinburgh. I often climbed Arthur's Seat and that summer I had taken a liking to hiking up to the top at dawn and meditating as the sun rose. On one of my many sleepless nights, however, I was a bit more adventurous.

I left my clothes at home and, saxophone in hand, I climbed to the top of Arthur's Seat. It was a cool, crisp night and it was invigorating to feel the cold air against my naked skin. It was delightful to feel the earth with my bare feet and to revel in the audacity of my endeavour. I didn't see anyone on the hill and played haunting improvised music to the night. I felt completely in tune with my authentic self. I was communicating directly with God; I felt more alive than ever before. I would recommend the experience to anyone!

I had a peculiar experience with one of my flatmates the next night. It was about 11.30pm and he was trying to talk to me. One of my other flatmates had vet exams coming up and had specifically asked me not to make any noise at nights. Holger was talking to me in the hall and very fixedly kept on talking. I wanted to say that I couldn't just stand there in the middle of the hall and talk to him because I'd promised Rachel that I wouldn't make any noise. For some reason I was unable to communicate that idea. It was essentially because when I was very high I developed a rather peculiar relationship with words. Whenever I uttered a word in that state, I had the feeling that the entire world changed, often dramatically. (Of course, in some sense the world does change with every word we utter, but normally we are not as conscious of that change as I was when I was high.) Only a few people seemed to be able to listen to what I had to say at those times without jumping to conclusions and generally misinterpreting what I was driving at.

In the end, after a few minutes of being 'rooted' in the hall by Holger, I decided that the only way I could get out of the situation was to turn my back and walk out of the front door. As I did so I was aware of dark, ominous symbols appearing in my aura. I ignored them and walked out of the flat and into the night. I later learnt that Holger had heard me swear at him angrily as I stormed out of the house. I realised then that what I was perceiving was very different to what the people around me were experiencing. My hypersensitivity to the interconnectedness of all things meant that every moment had to be carefully negotiated.

A few nights later I had another bizarre experience. This one was just before one of my visits to the Royal Edinburgh Hospital, and I really was in a pretty unusual state by this time, not having slept for days and days and probably not having taken my medication or eaten properly for a while either.

By studying maths I had developed my ability for abstract thought and found a particular affinity for geometric ideas. I loved the notion of points in high-dimensional spaces and often played with geometrical concepts in my mind.

I remember that for a few hours before the mind-blowing experience I'm about to describe, I had been attempting to visualise 4, 5 and higher dimensional spaces. I kept projecting sets of points onto different planes and imagining all sorts of weird and wonderful transformations of shapes. I worked faster and faster and could feel my mind limbering up as I progressed.

Suddenly I had an epiphany. It was similar in quality to my experience in 1995 when I read continuously for about 60 hours, but felt immeasurably more intense. I felt as though I had unlocked a door in my mind and I was open to receiving a new understanding of the world. I became aware of enormously evolved spiritual beings, who seemed to be playing some sort of game.

It was a game in which the definition of the pieces was part of the game. Thus the pieces were not necessarily simple 'objects'; rather, all boundaries between things dissolved and continuously shifting sets of impressions and regions of space-time were being manipulated by these unseen 'superbeings'.

At one point the dimensions of the flat flipped through some obscure transformation and the floor was now vertical. I became aware that the next 'move' in the game involved my moving from my room to the kitchen. It was like climbing a ladder to travel along the now-vertical floor. When

I reached the kitchen, reality snapped back into place and I was left with a feeling of 'This is what it's like on a higher level but you're not ready for it yet'. I was a person again, but a vastly enriched person with another mystical experience to my name.

May took me into hospital a few days later. There an even more bizarre set of perceptions hit me.

In the waiting room there was a chequerboard pattern on the floor. As we waited for me to be admitted to the ward I amused myself by playing the part of a queen, pawn or other playing piece on the chess board in front of me. May, to her credit, played along. It was a form of intellectual dance with both of us improvising a sequence of moves.

When ward 1 was ready for me I didn't feel like leaving the chess game I was playing in the waiting room. I could feel an electric charge beginning to build up and sensed that something interesting was about to happen.

Still wrapped up in my appreciation of 'The Game', I made my way, move by move, into the main concourse of ward 1. Then what started to happen was that the moves I was choosing to make conflicted more and more with what the hospital staff wanted of me. I was aware of my thoughts extending three or four feet above my head and they were buzzing like angry hornets. Coloured numbers began to flash above people's heads, with lower numbers for the patients and higher numbers for the nurses and doctors. One of the nurses 'scored' 6 while Professor Blackwood had a large 8 flashing above his head. I sensed that my own number was 9 but I was also aware of an invisible 'being' whose score was a staggering 23. This being along with some of its invisible helpers seemed to intervene from time to time to move people around and generally help to restore order in the rather confusing scene.

The nurses were scurrying around trying to keep me out of the way of the other patients as I moved seemingly erratically around the room, feeling 'The Game' coming to some sort of climax. Eventually I was held down by two security guards and injected with something to knock me out.

I remember nothing of the next four days although I was certainly conscious for some of that time. I learnt much later that May came in and gave me a bath at one point.

I wasn't in hospital for long that time – probably 10-14 days. But soon after I was released I was back into experimenting with consciousness, always pushing at the boundaries of perception.

I have labelled one of my experiences 'universal chiropractic'. In one of my meditation sessions I had asked the universe to provide me with the experience of opening up all seven of my chakras. The day after this prayer things started to happen that were fascinating and very obviously generated by my request. It began in the kitchen of my flat. There was a work surface next to the cooker and a shelf above it. At a certain moment I found myself leaning against the work surface when I felt a gentle force pushing me backwards. I didn't resist and I 'was moved' into a position in which the edge of the work surface was pressing into my lower back and my neck was resting on the shelf with my back inclined at an angle of about 45 degrees. There was then an audible click and I felt my vertebrae aligning.

I then left the flat and went for a walk in a park called The Meadows. What followed was a series of falls of increasing severity, with each one seeming to correspond to a higher chakra than the last.

For the third chakra I was walking along on the grass when I felt myself pushed backwards. Again I didn't resist and fell back straight onto the back of my head.

Landing on the grass was not too painful but the next time I was 'pushed over', I was on a street. I just let myself 'go with the flow' and landed with a bang on the concrete. I was alright but I decided then that there had to be an easier way to open myself to the universe. I didn't want to go through three more progressively more severe knocks. I cancelled my prayer and continued my walk.

The next thing that happened was that I began to hear voices. It was a bit like tuning in to different radio stations. I was aware that by tuning my inner ear I could pick up a range of commentaries on what was going on around me. Sometimes the voices seemed to be arguing with each other, mostly in incomprehensibly languages. I think that occasionally a phrase was in English but I don't remember at all what I heard. I had the impression that some of the voices were 'further out' than others as though they represented different levels of highly evolved beings. I was listening to a voice that was a long way out and I found myself walking straight towards a bus shelter. My feeling was that if I kept listening to the voice I would be able to walk straight through the glass. (There were other people on the street who may have been rather surprised had I succeeded!) At the last moment my awareness flipped to a different 'channel' and I swerved to miss the bus shelter. I later managed to convince myself that the only reason I didn't walk through the glass was because the people around me were not ready to witness it.

My friend Nadja visited me in hospital just after I had had these falling down experiences. She later told me about the enormous bumps I had on the back of my head when she met me in hospital. (I don't remember how she came to be feeling my head but somehow she did.)

That visit into hospital had a number of other notable features. I began to think about teleportation. Then suddenly everything around me seemed to involve teleportation and magic of one sort or another. I remember a wonderful scene in my room in hospital with Nadja. It seemed to me at the time that every star in the universe was a teleportation centre and that if we only knew how to harness the power of the stars we could instantly be transported to any point in the universe. I gradually broadened the notion to include anything that resembled a star even only slightly. There was a wooden cupboard in the room in the hospital. On the wood there were a number of markings; the wood had a speckled appearance. I vividly remember crouching in the cupboard with Nadja and discussing the possibility that every one of the 'eyes' on the wood's surface was a potential transportation point and that if one knew how, one could use the cupboard as a spaceship and travel anywhere in space or time.

Nadja has a well-developed spiritual and mystical side to her. She is now a doctor, but she maintains a healthy scepticism about Western medicine. She studied reiki and makes frequent use of it in her medical life. She was perfectly at ease talking with me about my wacky and peculiar ideas.

An Australian called Cameron moved into the boxroom of my flat that summer. He was an important influence on my life. He was very much into environmental issues and got me thinking about how I could change my life to reduce my environmental impact.

I was already reasonably environmentally aware when I met Cameron but when he arrived I was prompted to take environmental friendliness to new heights.

I kept adding to my idea of what it meant to live in tune with the environment until I got to the point where I decided to stop using any electricity at all. At that time I took cold showers and ate all my food raw. I was living on an organic, vegan diet and doing lots of daoist yoga (which involved visualising energy coursing round my body) and I felt fantastic.

Cameron was almost as clean-living as I was. He was a committed vegetarian who bought almost all his food from organic shops. He didn't drink alcohol and didn't smoke. He was also incredibly fit. He had spent seven years in Australia training with a dance troupe and was also skilled in acrobatics. During that summer he often joined me on early morning jaunts up Arthur's Seat, where we would meditate together at the summit.

There is a good story that comes from one of my early morning visits up Arthur's Seat that summer. I was alone on this occasion - Cameron may have moved out already by this time; he didn't live with me for very long. This particular experience took place very early. It was probably around 5am when I left my flat to hike up to the misty summit of Arthur's Seat. I sat at the top meditating for a while. As an amusing aside I will tell you what I was thinking about as I meditated atop the hill that morning. I'd recently entered a competition - some sort of free prize draw. The prize of the competition was going to be presented by the celebrity of your choice. At the time I really fancied Meg Ryan. So, as I sat at the top of Arthur's Seat, the sparkling city of Edinburgh all around me, I was desperately willing Meg Ryan into my life. I justified it as practising the New Age idea of manifestation. I felt that it was possible to use thought alone to attract any experience into one's life and I was hoping that by meditating on the idea of Meg Ryan every day for a while I would get to meet her and win the competition. Anyway, on this particular summer's morning, I went for a swim in one of the small lochs on Arthur's Seat after my meditation. The loch was icily cold and absolutely full of reeds. The reeds were a nuisance but the temperature was incredibly invigorating. I climbed out of the water, shook some of the water off myself and put on my shorts. My penis and testicles had fared the worst in the chilling water and felt rather numb at this point.

As I made my way round the hill on the road, I felt full of magic. I imagined that I was able to will things to happen by just thinking about it. I saw a couple of crows perching on the rocks. I decided to test my abilities. I looked at one of the crows and blinked at it, willing it to move. To my surprise and delight it did. As I repeated the experiment again and again it seemed to work every time. (Of course, crows are fickle creatures and don't like being looked at, but I genuinely believed I was willing them to keep flying on.) I decided to go for something bigger. I looked at the mass of rock that made up Arthur's Seat itself and decided to try to will it out of existence. (I'm not sure what would have happened to me had I succeeded, since I was on the hill myself, but that didn't bother me at the time.) I blinked repeatedly at the rock but failed to persuade it to disappear.

Undeterred by my failure to move mountains, I started running down the slope, heading back to my house. It was then that I experienced a novel sensation. I was suddenly aware that I was able to run very fast very easily. As my legs moved faster and faster, I reached a point where the world seemed to blur and I felt as though I was on the verge of accelerating to the speed of light. It was just as I tasted the hint of the infinite that I tripped and hit the ground very hard. The pain of striking the hard ground with my frozen genitalia was a very grounding experience. But I got up quickly and started to reflect on the experience. My interpretation of what had happened is an interesting one. I decided that I had attracted that particular experience in order to remind myself that our potential is unlimited, but that we are not ready for every experience at every moment. At no point did I think that it was impossible for me to run at speeds approaching the speed of light, but I did feel that I wasn't ready for those speeds just yet - it was as though I felt that I still had a lot of spiritual growing to do before I could really explore limitlessness.

I managed to maintain this extreme lifestyle for a few weeks; it was eventually stopped by yet another visit to hospital. The reasons for this hospitalisation may become apparent as you read some of the other things I was doing at the time.

The flat I'd moved into at the start of my second year of medicine in Parkside Terrace was witness to many of my manic episodes. During my time there I was often experimenting with social boundaries. One of these boundaries was the elusive notion of ownership. I basically stopped believing that it was possible to own anything, especially property. I enjoyed living in that flat so much that I was prepared to contemplate spending my entire life there. I therefore acted as though I was free to do whatever I wished with the flat although it was not technically mine. I did some things that really pushed the boundary of acceptability in terms of respect for other people's property.

In the kitchen in the Parkside Terrace flat there was a feature of plastic gold tiles. I knew that it was an aspect of the flat that the landlord particularly liked, however garish it seemed to most people. It was therefore an act of extreme disrespect for me to strip the tiles off the wall during one of my manic episodes without asking his permission. When I decided to put them on again I did so in two stages. Firstly I arranged the tiles in a mathematical pattern, putting in only those tiles that were in a prime number position (2, 3, 5,7,11, etc.), leaving spaces in the remaining places. I left that pattern up for a few days; I found it a very pleasing structure, appealing as it did to my aesthetic sense of number. However I eventually realised that it was not acceptable to leave the tiles like that so I finished off the job of retiling the wall. (My landlord almost never came round to the flat so he was never aware that I had stripped the tiles and put them back on again.)

There was a small storeroom close to the kitchen that was completely full of junk. The door was padlocked and we didn't have a key, but we could see through the frosted glass door and we could tell that the room was very full. As I applied feng shui principles to cleanse the flat I became more and more conscious of the heaviness of the junk in that storeroom. My cleansing had got to the stage where I was removing the doors of the flat to aid the flow of chi. I felt I had to do something about that heavy room. I broke open the padlock and set about disposing of all the stuff. Some of it was pretty bulky and I had to call the council to have the heavy items collected. There were a large number of bottles of home-made wine that looked as though they had been sitting there for decades. The wine went down the sink and I took the bottles to the recycling centre. When you consider that none of the stuff was mine and that it was in a room that I didn't even have access to you get some idea of how extreme my behaviour was. Amazingly my landlord took it very well when he found out that all his 'clutter' had been thrown away. The fact that I was taken to hospital very soon afterwards probably helped him to forgive my invasion of his privacy. I'm deeply grateful to him for being so understanding of my mental illness.

However unacceptable my behaviour was, it felt amazing once I had finished clearing out that room. It was as though the accumulated detritus had been weighing down the atmosphere of the flat. Once the storeroom was an active, usable space, the energy of the flat lifted dramatically.

My landlord had fitted blinds in my room. At some point the blinds got badly twisted and became almost unusable. I felt like having a light curtain to replace the ripped red curtains in my room. So, continuing to treat the flat as though I owned it, I removed the gnarled blinds and the old curtains and hung some light-coloured curtains. Once again it was only the fact that I was 'high' that meant my landlord could let me off.

As my energy levels rose, I felt less and less attached to material things. I started taking my stuff to charity shops in black bin-liners. As I cleared out more and more of my clutter I felt a fabulous lightening of my spirit.

I didn't stop giving my things away until I got down to two pairs of trousers and a few T-shirts. Apart from the piano and a few vases, I owned nothing. It was an extraordinarily liberating feeling.

The hardest things to get rid of were my clarinet and saxophone. When I came to thinking about clearing them out of my life I felt a lump in my throat. This was after all the clarinet I had asked my parents to send out to India by speed post when I realised I needed it to play with the National Symphony Orchestra of India. It was an instrument with history. The saxophone too had its story. I'd gone into a music shop with my parents as a sixteen-year-old thinking that I needed a new mouthpiece for my clarinet. The salesman had persuaded my parents that in fact I needed a new clarinet. He had a slightly battered saxophone he was trying to get rid of and, seeing my enthusiasm when he'd given me a go, he'd offered my parents a very reasonable deal for both instruments together. As I experienced a pang of anxiety at the thought of parting with my instruments, I immediately realised that these were the only two things I was genuinely attached to. I didn't hesitate; I immediately picked them up and walked out into the night. (During my clearing out phase I had very little sleep, and did a lot of work at nights, taking bags to charity shops and leaving them on the street outside.)

I ended up abandoning my musical instruments on the street outside a music shop. I remember justifying the decision to let go of my instruments by telling myself that I was just giving up particular instances of the clarinet and saxophone in favour of a more abstract, Platonic notion of the Clarinet and Saxophone as ideals. I felt at the time that there would come a time when I would play the instruments again; by stepping away from them for a while it would refresh my vision of music. I was playing jazz piano with a five-piece jazz band that summer. We played two or three times a week in a cafe in Edinburgh. Unfortunately I went into hospital in August. The band found a replacement pianist for a few weeks but then it dissolved.

During this period of my life my energy levels were higher than ever. I was talking furiously to anyone and everyone, baffling most people along the way. Dominic was the bass player from the jazz band. He was a fellow mathematician and helped me out on one occasion in particular by being a calm and unruffled listener who allowed me the space to talk about my thoughts in a non-judgmental way.

Dominic came round to my Parkside Terrace flat and found me high. We went out for a walk across town together. I was acting very strangely indeed and at a certain moment started pulling at Dominic's jacket and babbling senselessly. Dominic guided me through the streets to his own flat where he sat down and asked me to just talk.

It was a tremendously helpful conversation (albeit rather one-sided with me doing most of the talking). Dominic sat in a chair and listened and watched without saying anything as I used my whole being to communicate with him.

I danced around the room; I made huge, expansive gestures and kept up an uninterrupted stream of words in an attempt to put across my message. One idea I was working on involved thinking of each of us as a solid sphere, with our interactions occurring rather like balls colliding on the green felt of a pool table. I saw different people as differently coloured spheres of different densities, corresponding to their closeness to 'the source'.

As I gesticulated and danced wildly round Dominic's living room it felt like I was on a stage, finally having found an audience that was able to understand my message. There were no time constraints and Dominic just kept on listening until it was clear that I had finished my long monologue.

When I reached the end of my spiel he recommended a maths book to me that he said he thought was quite closely related to the ideas I was expressing. It was a book about a discipline called model theory. It was a very dense book and I only ever managed to get through the first two chapters. Still, Dominic was right that it was closely related to my own thinking. It talked about language (in a very abstract sense), logic and a mathematical notion of signatures. Maybe one day I will study model theory properly and genuinely understand what the book was about!

While I was playing with the jazz band in Cafe Dix-Neuf in Edinburgh I was in an elevated frame of mind most of the time. We were playing two or three times a week during the summer and I wasn't doing much else other than enjoying the summer sun. The band witnessed me going high and a visit into hospital prevented me from playing in the cafe during the festival in August.

On the day before I went into hospital in August 1999 I was playing with the band in the cafe. I often found that my playing loosened up significantly when I was high. At the time we had a singer with the band called Estelle. She had a gloriously powerful singing voice. Late in the evening one of the customers in the cafe asked the band for a particular song, whose title I forget. The only one of us who knew the song was Estelle and she agreed to sing it on her own.

As she started singing I decided I could probably improvise something to accompany her. The cafe owner, George, was suggesting that I have a go at accompanying a completely unfamiliar song. I would have given it a go were it not for the other band members, who, aware that I was a bit high and feeling that I had a super-inflated belief in my own abilities, strongly advised me against it. So in the end that opportunity passed me by.

The next day the band had arranged to come round to my flat for a rehearsal. When Dominic turned up, I was in the process of taking the doors of the flat off their hinges. I hadn't slept for a few days and I was in a fairly elevated frame of mind. The thinking behind removing the doors was to open the flat to the flow of energy in the spirit of feng shui.

One of the experiments I was doing at the time involved space. I was basically deliberately restricting the size of my world. The rationale for this was somewhat convoluted, but the idea was that I was an infinitely creative being and irrespective of how much of the world I explored I would only ever see a tiny fraction of it. So why not just stay in one place and fully appreciate every moment that came along? I had previously decided that there was no real need for me to leave Edinburgh and in the summer of 1999 I simply extended that idea and decided that there was no need for me to even leave my flat. I had plenty of food in the cupboards and a bowl full of money sitting on my desk.

When I said that I got rid of everything except for two pairs of trousers and two T-shirts I was not exaggerating - my renunciation of material possessions included throwing away my bank card, wallet and passport. One reason for throwing away my passport was that I had decided to just stay in Edinburgh and therefore had no need of a passport. Another reason was that I was aware that many people on Earth did not have the freedom to travel and by cutting myself off from the freedom that a passport offered I was empathising in some small way with the millions of people who were not free to travel. At the time I said to myself that I would live without a passport until the time when everyone on the planet could travel freely. I didn't stick to this philosophy for very long; I now have a passport again and enjoy travelling.

Dominic had come round without his instrument. The reason for this was that the previous evening when we had been playing in the cafe, it had been obvious to the other band members that I was going high. They realised that I would probably be in no state for a productive rehearsal the following day, but two of them came round to see how I was.

When the drummer arrived, I was sitting with Dominic in the kitchen of my flat, talking animatedly about the fabulous thoughts that were going through my mind. The front door of the flat was wide open (the kitchen was at the back of the flat). Sam, the drummer, was evidently very worried about me. He came into the kitchen and started talking about taking me to hospital. I gently refused his offer to take me to the Royal Edinburgh Hospital, stating that I was perfectly happy in the flat and had no need to leave. He then asked me for the name of my GP. I laughed and said that if Sam wanted to get me to hospital he would have to find out who my GP was by himself. I was enjoying the banter with Sam but he found it infuriating and soon left, on a mission to find my GP and get me into hospital. During my conversation with Sam, Dominic sat and listened. Afterwards he said that he could see what I was trying to do - I'd winked at him a few times during the conversation to show him that I wasn't actually all that serious about some of the things I said. Dominic and I carried on talking after Sam left.

Sam must have been successful since soon there came a knock at the still open front door. When I heard the knock I made no effort to go and answer the door. My doctor called 'hello' into the house, but I didn't budge. In the end Dominic got up and let my GP in. (I was just testing my GP - I was interested to see whether he was prepared to walk in through an open door. Clearly not!)

The doctor came into the kitchen. His aim was to get me into hospital and he offered to take me in his car. I politely refused, once again pointing out that I was perfectly happy in my own flat and had no need to leave. He tried hard to reason with me but I casually deflected each of his comments. I didn't feel like going into hospital so I simply sat tight.

Eventually he realised that he wouldn't be able to persuade me to leave the flat and he left to go and get a social worker. I don't know why he went to fetch a social worker but a while later he came back with a woman who was introduced as a social worker.

Again they had no luck in coaxing me to the psychiatric hospital so they soon scurried off to bring in reinforcements.

By the time the GP came round for the third time, this time accompanied by three policemen, Dominic had had to leave and I was in the flat on my own. When the police turned up I was once again in the process of unscrewing the hinges of one of the doors of the flat.

The police handled the situation extremely well. One of them offered to help me to remove the door, and had a go at unscrewing the extremely recalcitrant screws. After a while I lost interest in that project and went and sat at my piano. (When I've been high I have often found that my ability to improvise on the piano has been vastly improved. I'm sure that part of this has simply been a delusional change of perception, but it often felt easier to play than when I wasn't high.)

Having sat down to play I entered a trance-like reverie and let the notes tumble and cascade over one another. The policemen were standing at the door to my room, talking amongst themselves. A couple of times one of them came over to me and asked me if I would accompany them to the hospital. I didn't respond at all and simply carried on playing my music.

At a certain moment during my playing I had a feeling that it was nearly time for me to leave the house, and the next time a policeman came over to me I stopped playing, said something like 'Alright, let's go then' and walked out to the waiting police van.

Instead of doing anything as obvious as sitting on one of the benches in the back of the police van, I stretched myself out horizontally between the two benches and lay in this difficult position for a short while. I couldn't maintain it all the way to the hospital and changed to sitting in a full lotus meditation pose on the floor of the vehicle.

The police first took me to the wrong hospital. We arrived at the Royal Infirmary which is not a psychiatric hospital. One of the policemen went inside, only to discover that they were in the wrong place.

While he was gone, I had a delightful experience. I look out of the window of the van and saw the leaves of a sycamore tree outlined against a cloudless blue sky. The amazing part of the vision was the startlingly clear energy field I could see surrounding each leaf. Each leaf was contained in a pulsating, bright white aura that reminded me of images produced by Kirlian photography.

The police finally succeeded in getting me to the right hospital. After a brief show of not intending to leave the van, I allowed myself to be guided into ward 1; back among old friends.

I was in hospital for at most a couple of weeks on that occasion. I came out some time in the middle of August. My birthday is August 27th, and as I was 25 that year I decided to have a party. I settled on the theme of 'Jazz and Cheese' and invited lots of people round to my flat. I asked everyone to bring something beginning with the first letter of their name; James brought jalapeno peppers, Jemima brought jelly beans and Cameron provided a couple of cheeses that began with C. But the gift that best fitted with the empty, chi-filled flat came from Nicola. She presented me with an empty cardboard box and told me that it was a box of neutrinos. I laughed joyfully as I received her present. The party was a great success and a tremendous end to the summer.

A month or two after giving away everything I owned in Edinburgh I went home to visit my parents. I had by that time decided that the time had come for me to reintroduce things into my room. There were plenty of books, clothes and other items of mine at my parents' house and I filled as many bags as I could carry for my journey back to Edinburgh. It was the most heavily laden trip I've ever made.

On the train on the way up to Edinburgh I sat and talked to a woman who had made some extraordinary hitchhiking journeys across Europe. The idea of giving away all one's possessions did not strike her as strange at all; she had lived with minimal possessions at various times in her life. As I sat and chatted I felt a strong desire to simply abandon all the stuff that I had with me on the train and to carry on living with nothing. I mentioned it to my travelling companion, who smiled wryly. In the end I did cart all my stuff off the train with me, but the temptation was there.

Somehow I made it to my Edinburgh flat with all my bags. The floor of my room was completely covered with my things when a friend came round to give me some money he owed me. It was a total of £200 and I decided to go out on a shopping trip.

I went to the university James Thin bookshop and a large WHSmiths and managed to spend £200 on books without any trouble. I was feeling quite tired so I also bought some homeopathic sleeping tablets from Boots.

It was as though I had swung from wanting to get rid of everything in my life to wanting to accumulate as much in the way of material goods as possible.

At this stage I was thinking in terms of spinning thoughts about abstract axes in a geometric way. At one point this created an interesting and unusual conversational scenario.

I went round to May's flat. May wasn't in but I spoke to her flatmates for a while. I was very high.

One thing I was doing was collapsing time in my mind. I never wear a watch and have never really believed in time. What I did that day was to define a `Kim-moment'. I asked May's flatmates to time ten minutes on their watches and tried to explain that everything that took place during that period constituted the first ever recorded Kim-moment. During those ten minutes I danced around madly, conversing effervescently and generally behaved in what must have seemed a very peculiar fashion.

One of May's flatmates, a New Zealander called Helen, felt sufficiently worried about me to want to try to take me to hospital.

As Helen and I left May's flat we began a sort of dance with me trying to find a way to evade being taken to hospital. At first Helen didn't know which hospital to take me to. When she realised I needed to be taken to the Royal Edinburgh Hospital we started walking in that general direction. However, the Royal Ed is a long way from May's flat and as I was not in a mood to be taken to hospital and Helen had no experience of taking me into hospital, we never made it. Helen eventually agreed to leave me sitting on a park bench; she had to go to work and didn't really have time to walk me all the way to the psychiatric hospital. The conversation I alluded to earlier was a conversation that Helen and I had about minimalism as we wandered in the vague direction of the hospital.

Helen had come over from New Zealand and was living a relatively spartan existence in the boxroom of May's flat. She considered herself a minimalist. I too considered myself a minimalist, and 'minimalism' became the 'axis' about which I began rotating my thoughts.

Helen found it difficult to reconcile my statement that I was a minimalist with the fact that I had just returned from my parents' house absolutely laden down with stuff. However, it was pointless trying to reason with me in the state I was in. As we spoke my definition of minimalism kept broadening as I spun it round and round in my head. I was reflecting the concept of minimalism in the mirror of consumerism while simultaneously thinking about rotating New Zealand and travel about some other obscure axis in my mind. These exciting thoughts and my high levels of energy meant that I was leaping around maniacally as we moved erringly towards the hospital.

A few days later, May took me into hospital. I remember a strange experience just as we were about to leave May's flat for yet another hospitalisation. A male friend of May's, whom she'd lived with in the flat that was broken into, was in the flat at the time. He was a sparky, playful computer scientist who shared May's passion for word games and puzzles. I suppose the fact that he wasn't emotionally attached to the situation helped him to take an objective observer's perspective. Anyway, I realised as I was flying around May's kitchen, expressing my sheer delight at being alive, that this friend of May's was making more eye contact with me than any of the other people in the room were. He looked at me when I was speaking, and used his eyes to great effect to smile at my jokes and reassure me that he was not judging me in any way.

It was an event that contributed to my understanding of just how powerfully it is possible to communicate with our eyes alone. As I made eye contact with him, I recognised a kindred spirit, a fellow amused traveller on the comedic stage of this thing called mortal life. I had no time to savour that eye contact, since May was desperately trying to bundle me out of the flat and get me off to hospital, but it stayed with me.

As I looked into his eyes and realised the playfulness that was hidden in them, I started imagining how much fun it would be to play some sort of game with this guy. All I could fit in the hubbub of the action-packed scene was

"Chess, my place, some time!"

Which I said pretty loudly and very quickly. As I expected, a glint appeared in his eye as he smiled back. (Although we never played that game of chess, I love the cosmic significance that its potentiality took on for me.)

Another time Simon and James took me into hospital. It was after an event in a graveyard that Simon found extremely shocking. I include his account of that in the appendix. I stayed with Simon in James' flat for a time while James did some errands. I remember eating an entire banana, skin and all, just as a sensory experiment. One common feature of a lot of my manic episodes was a desire to experience things I had never experienced before. (Playing my saxophone naked at the top of Arthur's Seat was a classic example.)

When I arrived on Ward 1 that day I greeted the residents with my usual flamboyance and joyfulness. A lot of the faces were familiar to me from my previous visits to the hospital.

After a round of colourful introductions I went into the kitchen of the ward and decided to use the entire room as a canvas for a 'painting'. Instead of paints, I used whatever I could lay my hands on - salt, sugar, bread, butter and the chairs and tables. I set to rearranging the dining area of the ward kitchen into a massive scale piece of abstract art. It felt amazing to be living creatively, utterly absorbed in the task. But for me, the most entertaining aspect of that incident was when one of the nurses came into the kitchen and, witnessing what I had done, ordered me to put the kitchen back exactly as I'd found it. Taking her words literally, I set to, relishing the creative challenge of restoring the furniture and decoratively employed foodstuffs to the positions they were in when I arrived in the room. I began the task with phenomenal energy and ebullience, but the nurse soon told me to stop what I was doing and leave the kitchen.

It was during that stay in hospital that I produced some of my most wild and cathartic works of art. We had regular occupational therapy sessions, when we would often do practical, artistic activities. My friend Holger came to visit me in hospital that time and together we painted an extraordinarily vivid and textured painting on a huge piece of linen-like material. I used only red and green paint. When I looked at the picture later I felt that it resembled the Turin Shroud. Without intending to, it seemed to me that I had painted an image of Christ as he was when he died. It seemed appropriate, somehow.

Another time in hospital, I was convinced that people were somehow transforming into each other, or 'morphing' as I called it. I believed that NASA had discovered some fantastic technology that enabled people to spin round a pole and turn into someone else. One of the male nurses in the hospital had very short hair, like my friend Cameron, and for a long time I didn't see Cameron and this nurse together, so I concluded that Cameron was secretly turning into this nurse in order to keep an eye on me even when he didn't seem to be around. (Cameron was training to be a nurse at the time so he would not have been out of place in a hospital setting.)

There were three nurses in the hospital at the time who reminded me of people I knew. As well as the nurse who reminded me of Cameron, there were also two others - a woman who looked a bit like Gemma and another who looked a bit like Maria - the Polish woman I got engaged to. It was very confusing in that tortured mental state to have people around me who so vividly resembled important women in my life. I actually took the nurses to one side one day and asked them if they were in fact Gemma and Maria. It felt good to imagine that Gemma and Maria were nearby;

maybe I was subconsciously expressing the fact that I wanted to see them both.

It was that same episode when two of the other patients in the hospital made a particular impression on me. Both men were a lot older than me. My grandfather had recently died and it seemed to me that each of the two patients embodied some aspect of my grandfather's side of the family. As I spoke to the elder of the two men, I had the impression that he was a brother or uncle of my deceased grandfather. He looked a bit like my grandfather and had enormous, bushy eyebrows. His appearance reminded me of an owl and as I had collected owls as a child I felt that he had chosen this particular appearance to help me recognise him as a relative. I imagined in my mania that at nights this old man would somehow fall out of the hospital window and turn into an owl, returning to the hospital the following morning after a night on the wing. He seemed to protect me at times. When I ventured into the smoking lounge where the piano was, it seemed that Owlman kept an eye out for me. When I tried to initiate conversation with one of the deeply embittered old patients, Owlman would step in and smooth the ruffled feathers of the old vulture when I revealed something inappropriately personal or otherwise failed to sense the social etiquette of the older patients.

The other patient who left an indelible impression on me was the Wordmaster. He reminded me of my father's brother although the Wordmaster was probably at least 15 years older than my uncle. The Wordmaster had studied Greek and Latin at school and seemed to have a tremendous grasp of English grammar, including the names of all sorts of obscure parts of speech such as copula and adjunct. The thing that particularly impressed me about the Wordmaster was his ability to have loads of different conversations simultaneously. If he was speaking to someone and someone else interrupted, he would acknowledge the new speaker and continue both conversations. Sometimes this was extended to five or six simultaneous exchanges. The most extraordinary thing was that I had the sensation that he was speaking in different colours to the different people in the conversations. I perceived his different modes as different shades of grey and brown. It was surreal but very interesting to be perceiving such unusual things in my altered state.

Kim Evans

Helen: Ribbons of Thought

In about May 1999 I met Helen, a medic whom I feel great fondness for. (Note that this is not the same Helen as the woman from New Zealand who lived with May.) She was witness to various attempts on my part to annihilate my Self. When I met her, I was grappling with notions of identity. My thinking was influenced by the fact that I was studying mathematics by that time. Mathematics is a discipline in which the idea of identity is commonplace. Obviously the words *identity* and *identical* have the same root, and a lot of mathematics is about establishing whether two or more seemingly different objects are in fact the same. This was the motivation for my exploration of the concept of identity. I was particularly fascinated by the idea of reflections somehow preserving the identity of the thing being reflected.

I met Helen at a musical charity event organised by another medic friend, Nadja. I immediately liked Helen. She had a very individual look, with spiky hair and clothes that stood out from the crowd. At the end of the evening I walked home with her and had a drink at her house.

I rapidly fell in love with Helen and, as a result of her not wishing to go out with me coupled with my inability to deal intelligently with my emotions, I spiralled helplessly out of control and landed myself in hospital within a fortnight of meeting her. In the run up to my hospitalisation, I tried desperately to erase myself - it was as though I wanted to have nothing to do with the Kim Evans of the past. I wanted to dissolve into a sea of Nirvana.

I've had many fascinating conversations with Helen over the last few years. She has visited me in hospital on numerous occasions and she has seen me very high indeed and hardly batted an eyelid.

When I first met Helen and immediately started to go high, I was exploring the notion of reflection. I would have a thought and then try to imagine what that thought would be if it were reflected in some abstract plane or rotated about a particular axis. The planes and axes I defined in my mind were constructed from words and images and didn't consist of anything that had any genuine mathematical meaning. For example, I might see a bird and imagine rotating the thought of that bird about an axis made by connecting the concepts 'honesty' and 'truth'. There was an unnerving wildness to my thinking during this period - I was flying rapidly from abstraction to abstraction and I was in a state that made it almost impossible for me to concentrate on my studies.

One of the 'reflectors' I developed most was eyes. Here the idea of reflection was much less abstract, in that when we look into somebody's eyes we genuinely do see a reflection of ourselves. And our reflection has eyes that reflect the world outside and so on ad infinitum. I started to imagine what all the reflections looked like in all the eyes of the animals and people I encountered. The 'real world' rapidly dissolved into an infinite array of reflected images. It was as though I had converted my perceptual filter into a sort of kaleidoscope; I was now revelling in the myriad subtle patterns of light that danced around between our minds and reflective surfaces. One evening as I was still on the way up, I went to see Helen in her flat. She was doing a life-drawing of one of her flatmates. The television was on in the background. At a certain moment a picture appeared on the screen in which the screen was split into lots of small images with each one containing a person's face. I felt myself reflected in all of the eyes on the screen; it was as though I was a glass vessel that had been smashed into hundreds of tiny pieces while still maintaining some sort of unity. The fragmentation of self was an exhilarating experience and I felt a desire to lose myself further and to explode outwards in every direction possible at the speed of light, like a Big Bang.

I wanted to become something else, to cut all ties with the image of Kim Evans I had been projecting all my life. I felt an intense desire to change absolutely everything about myself - to shave my head or dye my hair blue, to mutate into an albatross or a dolphin, to be everything simultaneously. I asked Helen if I could have a shower. She said later that I was in the shower for an incredibly long time. I think I spent a lot of the time gazing at the reflection of myself in my eyes in the mirror and enjoying the dancing patterns of light in the room.

I don't remember exactly how I got into hospital that time, but Helen certainly came to visit me frequently and I remember having long conversations about the great Conversation of Life. I was still thinking about eyes and viewed every eye movement and every blink or wink as an exchange in a multilayered Conversation that everything was engaged in. I thought of eyeballs as a kind of memory for particular 'phrases' in this multidimensional Conversation. It was an intense and often sleepless time. Interestingly the antipsychotic drugs I was given only served to heighten the intensity of my focus on eyes. I say this because the drugs seemed to enable me to see the unity of all things more easily. When I was taking the drugs, my vision was affected. My ability to sharply focus diminished; the world seemed to blur. I became exceedingly aware of the pupils of people's eyes. I felt sucked into the gaping pools of blackness.

Helen witnessed some other strange things that I did. These were all in the same manic episode.

One evening, Helen and I went to see a play at the Traverse Theatre in Edinburgh. I was still very much trying to shed my self. As we waited in the queue I took my wallet out of my pocket and proceeded to discard all of the pieces of identification I had on me. By the time we arrived in the theatre I no longer had any form of ID on me; all my cards were simply lying on the floor of the corridors of the theatre.

During the performance there was someone on stage signing the show for deaf people. I was in a funny state of mind and got so caught up in the movements that the signer was making that I began making similar movements in response. It is probably just as well we were right at the back of the theatre since otherwise I may have rather disrupted the performance. Soon afterwards I was again in hospital.

Another time I was with Helen in a pub. The way I have described what was going on in my thoughts at this time is like a three-dimensional ticker tape. There was a square window in the centre of my mind and all my thoughts were on long ribbons that passed through the window as I thought them.

I was in an extremely energetic and elevated state. What I was focusing on in the pub that day was double letter combinations. What this meant was that whenever a word containing a double letter passed through the central window of my mind, I would immediately switch onto a different ribbon of thought that also contained that same double letter combination. So for example, if I was thinking the thought 'There is an apple on the table', the thought would break apart at the double 'p' and I might continue (in either direction) with the thought 'Happy are those who love' from the double letter in that thought. The transitions were instantaneous - I was able to generate suitable sentences without any hesitation; it requires a bit of thought when I'm not high.

There was a central wall in the pub that it was possible to walk all the way round. At one point I took it into my head to run round the room whenever I encountered a double letter combination in my thinking. I thus became a sort of whirling dervish, frenetically charging round the room at incomprehensible moments (incomprehensible, that is, to the people watching!)

Helen was amazing during these times. She supported me both in and out of hospital and allowed me enormous freedom to be myself, not trying to rein me in. Helen was never involved in the process of putting me into hospital. That role fell predominantly to May and James.

Interlude: New Age Literature

This is as good a moment as any to mention the 'Conversation with God' books that played a very important formative role in my thinking.

May bought book 1 for me shortly after I changed from medicine to maths. The author is Neale Donald Walsh. The books are presented as a dialogue between the author and God. Book 1 concerns personal issues; relationships, money, Who We Really Are, what God is like and other themes. The basic idea is that God wants to communicate the idea that there are no absolute rights and wrongs and that the whole purpose of life is self-definition and creation. We are one with God and God communicates with everyone at all times. God is trying to dispel the notion that we need any intermediaries (such as priests) to interpret God's messages for us; by listening to our hearts we can all communicate with God directly.

Once I had read book 1 I was hooked. I read and reread it and waited eagerly for books 2 and 3 to come out. (They covered the geopolitical situation and the journey of the soul respectively.) Through my reading I cultivated a keen awareness of my own limitlessness and this is what I was expressing through my crazy actions.

Another feature of the Conversations with God series is the idea that there is no such thing as coincidence. Everything happens for a reason and there is perfection in every moment. A consequence of this, when coupled with our own soul awareness, is that we each attract into our lives exactly the right set of experiences for our particular life path. There is perfect reciprocity in that every action by one soul towards another is taking place according to some pre-arranged 'contractual' agreement between those souls. Thus it is not possible to do something to another that is against their will; we cannot impose anything on anyone else. If one accepts this powerful and liberating notion then even situations where one soul *appears* to be imposing their will on another can be understood in a different way as two perfect life paths interacting. Thus some souls choose paths that include violence, terror or pain and suffering as part of their spiritual growth. And growing through suffering is one way to proceed in life, though there are certainly other routes to growth - suffering is unnecessary.

The incident with the bus shelter when I failed to walk through glass reminds me of a scene from the book 'Jonathan Livingstone Seagull' by Richard Bach. The story is about a seagull (Jonathan), who has no interest in living the humdrum, food-centred lifestyle of his flock, but rather wishes to devote his life to learning how to fly perfectly. At a certain point, Jonathan has returned to his flock in order to guide other aspiring flyers to mastery. He is leading a group of students through an aerobatic stunt when a young gull from the flock flies in front of one of the speeding students. The speeding gull veers sharply to avoid the young one, and collides with the sheer and unyielding surface of a cliff. To his surprise, the voice of The Great Gull (Jonathan), addresses him and informs him that flying through solid rock is a more advanced stage of the program than the student is currently ready for. Jonathan offers the gull the opportunity to return to the flock and the student wakes up at the bottom of the cliff, much to the astonishment of the watching flock.

(It is the notion of an ever-advancing program of challenges that is relevant here; there's not much of a link between Jonathan bringing the gull back to life and my failing to walk through a bus shelter!)

MEMORIES OF MANIA

First attempt at finishing a degree

In September 1999, May and I redecorated the Parkside Terrace flat (this time with the landlord's permission). In the space of a few weeks we transformed the place, making the kitchen a brightly coloured and welcoming room and whitewashing the rest of the flat. My landlord even paid me for the work. It meant that my last year in that flat was particularly enjoyable as every day I beheld the fruits of my labour. Surprisingly, when I moved out of that flat the landlord told me I was the best tenant he'd ever had. This was in spite of my having done things to his property that were probably illegal and certainly disrespectful.

I got a job in October of 1999, working 15 hours a week as a French teacher in a nursery. It was one of the most enjoyable jobs I have ever done. I worked with 3-5 year olds and, using games, songs and other activities, succeeded in teaching them some basic French.

The first semester of my fourth year of maths was a lot of fun. One of the courses I particularly enjoyed was a mathematical education module. It involved going into primary schools in groups of three and teaching the children about three-dimensional shapes. When it came to writing up the report over the Christmas holidays I decided to write mine in a rather creative way. I did the writing by hand with a beautiful calligraphy pen and included various paintings in my report. I used the metaphor of travelling in a space ship to

149

colonies in a far-off galaxy. The children were the colonists and their teachers were colony leaders. It was a fabulous way to write. I hope it gave the person marking the course as much pleasure to read as I gained from writing it.

In March 2000 things began to get difficult again. I think it may have been because I was doing almost exclusively statistics modules in the second semester of that year, and felt that there was a whole body of pure maths underlying the statistical ideas that I was missing out on. I couldn't bear the idea of finishing my degree without having had the chance to study the modules I wanted to and I think this tension was part of what triggered my mania on this occasion. I ended up resitting the final year of my degree, and second time round I changed my degree from maths and statistics to pure mathematics. That meant that I was not obliged to take a certain number of statistics modules and could really concentrate on the pure mathematics. I got through that second attempt at fourth year with only one visit to hospital. It was altogether better than the first time round.

I remember a day at the nursery a few days before I went into hospital. I was in a state of mind in which I felt an amazing sense of connection and, possibly delusional, I felt that I had the power to influence the behaviour of inanimate objects. At one point we were attempting to show the children a video of a French cartoon. The picture was rather fuzzy.

Wanting to give the children the best experience possible, I stood perfectly still and attempted to 'tune in' to the functioning of the television and video. I tried to use my mind to hold the picture steady so the children could watch the film. Obviously I was somewhat preoccupied during this time and my quietness was noticed by the manager of the nursery.

Another event of that day at the nursery involved playing with a child who was winding a piece of string around a toy. The toy was a set of metal 'tracks' with different coloured beads on, which presented plenty of opportunity to get the string into very complicated patterns. The way I was thinking that day I was very much in a non-intervention mood. I let the girl carry on playing with the string until it was completely snarled up around the metal pieces. The manager came round and said it was time to pack things away. The girl didn't want to just cut the string so together we set about disentangling the strands. It was a delightful exercise to watch her dealing with a very complicated problem (she was four). Eventually we ran out of time and had to resort to scissors. During the time that I had been sitting with the girl we had both been utterly absorbed in the activity. We were both in 'the zone', enjoying a timeless sense of wonder at our engagement with the problem.

I was full of energy at the time (a common feature of my manic episodes). I felt as though I was fuelled by some infinite source of exuberance and joy. I ended up in hospital a few days later. The manager of the nursery came round to see me as did lots of my friends.

I had received a letter a short while before my hospitalisation that may well have contributed to my going high. When I started working at the nursery I was supposed to have a police check. However, because the manager of the nursery needed someone urgently, I started working before the check had been completed. It took until March before the result came back. I received a letter from Edinburgh Council informing me that it had been decided that I was not allowed to work with children under eight. Since I really loved working at the nursery, I should have let myself feel the disappointment associated with receiving the letter. Instead, my feelings emerged in the form of another visit to hospital.

After a week or so in the hospital in Edinburgh my parents decided to come and collect me and take me back to their house. It was there, in the run-up to Easter 2000, that some very dramatic events took place.

Almost as soon as I arrived at my parents' house I felt a desire to leave and to return to Edinburgh. I had no money and was not in a state in which I wanted to use money. One day, early in the morning, I went outside to our barn. I took my father's bike, intending to cycle all the way to Edinburgh (about 300 miles).

As I headed north I felt an extraordinary sense of freedom. It felt amazing to have 'stolen' my father's bicycle and to be on my way back to Edinburgh. I was cycling on the towpath next to the canal about two miles from my parents' house when the speedometer on my dad's bike began to get on my nerves. I found that having numbers continuously flashing at me distracted my attention from appreciating the beautiful scenery around me and simply enjoying the ride. My solution was to remove it and throw it by the side of the path. (At this point I should say that throughout my childhood I was always very keen to please my parents - I always respected them and never rebelled. The act of discarding my father's speedometer, knowing that he liked having it, illustrates how peculiar a state of mind I was in. It did feel exciting to rebel in this small way!)

I got as far as Burton-on-Trent - an eight mile ride. It was still early and the streets were extremely quiet. I was riding round the town centre, often on the 'wrong' side of the street or on the pavements. I was breaking the rules that previously I had adhered to with military precision.

I rode into a car park and rode round and round. To give you some idea of my state of mind, at one point I decided to attempt to ride *through* a lamppost. I viewed it as an investigation of the properties of the material world. If Jesus walked on water, I reasoned, then surely I can ride a bike through a solid object. I wasn't going particularly fast when I hit the lamp post - just fast enough to give my balls a short sharp jolt of pain as they collided with the crossbar. No miracles that day!

Needless to say, I was not really in the right state of mind for the sustained focus necessary for a 300 mile cycle ride. I pottered around Burton town centre for a while, waiting for the shops to open. I was getting hungry but I had no money. However, I must have had some sort of ID with me, because when the banks opened I was able to go into my branch and withdraw the money I had left, which amounted to about £1.50. I remember going into Sainsbury's and buying some doughnuts. It was a symbolic moment; for a long time I had had no money and had been unable to purchase anything. Finally I was able to use my own money to buy something again.

I decided that I would go on the train to Edinburgh instead of cycling. The only problem with that idea was my lack of money. But I did have my father's bike. I decided to try and sell it to generate enough money for the train fare. I went into a bike shop and asked about the possibility of their buying the bike. Fortunately they refused. By this time I was beginning to find the bike a bit of a burden and ended up simply leaving it at the front of the shop and walking unencumbered onto the street. I still felt like getting on a train so I did, disregarding the fact that I had no ticket. I didn't get very far. The conductor came round to check tickets pretty promptly. When he discovered that I had neither a ticket nor the means with which to buy one he phoned ahead to the station police at

Derby. I was in a state in which I didn't really differentiate between different places or times and attempted to initiate a conversation with the conductor about the non-existence of trains and the freedom of space and time.

When we arrived in Derby the station police were ready for me. When I realised that I was not going to make it to Edinburgh I left the train and after initially walking away from the police I eventually accepted that I couldn't get out of the situation and went with them to their office.

As I was sitting in the police office in Derby station I felt a fabulous sense of timelessness that has been repeated during many of my manic episodes. I was completely indifferent to the outside world and totally absorbed in the moment. I engaged in lively banter with the police woman who had shown me into the office and I felt great.

After obtaining my parents' details the police rang my parents and told them what had happened. I spoke to my father and told him where his bike was. My father said that he would come and collect me.

Half an hour later my father arrived in Derby train station. Both he and my mother had been extremely worried about me and obviously believed that I was very high indeed. My father was armed with six chlorpromazine tablets (we have since argued about exactly what dose they were, but I'd certainly never taken six at once before.)   Chlorpromazine is a powerful antipsychotic drug with lots of unpleasant side effects. My father insisted that I take all six tablets and then took me home.

Within about half and hour of arriving at my parents' house I was beginning to feel distinctly unwell. At first my parents ignored my telling them I felt sick, but soon I was flat on my back on the bathroom floor with both of my parents looking on with concern. It felt as though I was falling into a huge, black abyss. My heart was slowing down and I seemed to be losing touch with the world. At a certain moment, after taking a breath, my heart actually stopped beating. My mother, who was taking my pulse at the time, gave a shriek and immediately bent over to give me mouth to mouth resuscitation and ordered my father to ring for an ambulance. But as my mother's mouth met mine I simply exhaled and my heart restarted. The long, lingering moment of sweet emptiness was over, only to be replaced with much more frenetic times.

The ambulance arrived and I was raced off to a hospital in Burton-on-Trent. I don't remember much of the next few hours as I was nursed back to health. My impressions of that period are a confused jumble of images, with people coming and going from my bedside. When I was well again I was moved to the psychiatric hospital where I spent a couple of weeks.

When I later recounted the story to my friends, I pointed out that for someone who thought of himself as Christ to 'die' in Lent of 2000 was rather appropriate. My mother told me a story about what happened when we arrived at the hospital. When she gave my details to the man on reception he asked whether I had a twin called Christon. The hospital records had me down both as Kim Evans and as Christon Jan Evans. My mother explained that the two were the same person and said it was alright to 'kill' the Christon record.

As you can see from reading this, even at this stage, five years after my initial hospitalisation, the 'Christ theme' had not gone away. It was an extremely compelling story I was creating for myself - the idea that I had the potential to be the Second Coming and bring about global harmony was extraordinarily beguiling and hard to let go of.

Soon I was out of hospital and went back up to Edinburgh to continue with my maths degree. I was in the final year of the degree but I didn't end up graduating in 2000.

I was hospitalised a few more times between Easter and June and my study was so disrupted that there was no way that I could sit my exams that year. I spoke to my Director of Studies, who agreed that it made no sense for me to sit my exams after so much illness. I decided to return to university in September and resit my fourth year.

During the summer of 2000 I got a job as an English teacher on a summer school for Italian students near Cork. It was a situation that allowed me to be fairly high the whole time; one could argue that a touch of hypomania is very useful when managing groups of boisterous Italian teenagers.

One of our duties at the summer school was meeting the Italians off the plane in Cork airport. On the day I went to the airport I had just had an injection of clopixol - another antipsychotic that is given in reasonably severe cases of mania. The drug affected me a great deal, leaving me with a heavy, lethargic feeling and a dull pain behind my eyeballs.

The plane we were waiting for was delayed and didn't turn up until about 2am. I felt desperately groggy and needed sleep. I couldn't get comfortable in the airport seats. It was certainly the least pleasurable experience of the summer job.

By the time the summer school had finished I had managed to save about £900. I was feeling good about myself and was looking forward to returning to my maths study.

When I restarted at Edinburgh in October, I chose a completely new set of modules, with much more emphasis on pure maths than statistics. It felt fabulous to be studying delightfully abstract concepts. I spent a lot of time helping other people on the course with the coursework. I was in my element.

Moving House

I moved out of my Parkside Terrace flat in July 2000, at the end of my first attempt at the fourth year of the maths degree. During August and early September 2000, I stayed with Cameron, my Tasmanian friend, for a couple of weeks while I searched for a new place to live. I succeeded in finding a room in a wonderful five-bedroomed flat close to the maths department.

The flat was on a road called Ross Gardens. The other people living there were Alec, Mike, Richard and Sebastian. They were studying philosophy, chemistry, astrophysics, and meteorology with business studies respectively.

I met Mike first. When I first arrived at the flat I needed to go to Sainsbury's to do some food shopping. Mike immediately volunteered to accompany me; I liked him straight away.

I had lots of interesting conversations with Alec, the philosophy student, over the course of the year. His views were a little more materialist than mine, meaning that he believed in the existence of the world whereas I didn't, so there was plenty for us to discuss.

As far as my maths degree was concerned, I was yet again with a totally new group of people, having been into hospital so many times the previous year that I had to resit my final year. The change from a maths and statistics degree to a pure maths degree suited me. The constraint of having had to do five statistics modules the previous year had been a contributory factor in my going high so many times.

I have not stayed in touch with any of the people I met when I dropped back a year and changed to pure maths. I already had a well-established and supportive group of friends and although I got on well with some of the people on the course, I was not really with them long enough to build friendships that lasted. Having said that, I initially only met Gemma for four weeks when I first arrived at Queens' College but I have stayed in touch with her. Somehow the people on the maths course just didn't grab my attention enough for them to become lifelong friends. My mental state was stable until Easter of that year (2001). By then the second semester had started and the final exams were fast approaching.

Mary: How we met

In March 2001 I started going out with another girl. Once again her name was almost the name of someone close to Jesus but this didn't particularly feature in my thinking. This time I'm going to use the name Mary. She was living with a girl on my course, and I met Mary at a party that was organised by one of the other people on the maths course.

The party was a porn party. It was a splendid place to meet a future girlfriend. The organisers had gone to a huge amount of effort. A four-foot papier mache penis with accompanying cannon-ball sized testicles hung brazenly from the ceiling. The nozzles of the wine boxes were poking through cardboard cutouts of male upper torsos, giving the impression that the wine was coming out of the penises of the cutouts. Silhouettes of Bond-style dancing girls made from black paper lined the walls of the front bedroom. In the same room the furniture had been removed and replaced with a huge paddling pool lined with leopard-print cushions. Another room had been set up as a 'fist of fun cinema', with a range of pornographic films showing all night. The costumes of the people at the party were great, with a lot of the men sporting chest wigs and enormous gold medallions. One of the people who lived in the flat had bought a PVC nurse's outfit especially for the occasion. I wore a kimono. My only rationale for choosing to wear a kimono to a porn party was that it could be the sort of thing that porn stars would slip on between filmings.

I got talking to Mary fairly early on in the evening and I was immediately impressed by her unusual sense of humour and her sense of fun. (She had not dared to dress in a pornographic way so there was no 'stage persona' to deal with.) She was studying German and Swedish at the time and we talked about her experiences of spending time in both Germany and Sweden between her third and fourth years of study. She seemed open, witty and warm-hearted, and by the end of the evening we were hugging and kissing in the paddling pool, everyone else having conveniently vacated the room.

I thoroughly enjoyed getting to know Mary. She was lively and fun to be with. Our first date was to see the film 'Chocolat' and we just carried on from there. Mary had been a very diligent student during her time in Edinburgh and hadn't really explored what the city had to offer in terms of restaurants, cinemas and entertainment in general. It was great to show her places she had never seen before.

Falling in love is a well-documented trigger for hypomanic episodes. When I went high at Easter of my final year, being in love was probably one of the factors. However, there was something else that happened that also destabilised me a bit.

A Disappointing Letter Leads to Derailment

I was starting to think about what I wanted to do after finishing my maths degree. The idea of teaching in secondary schools held a great deal of appeal. Both of my parents have been teachers at some point in their lives and I had enjoyed all the teaching work I had done in the past; it seemed a perfectly natural choice. I applied for a place at Exeter University to study for a PGCE.

The interview in Exeter went extremely well and I received a letter informing me that I had a place on the maths PGCE course. However, a few weeks later, after my health check had been completed, I received a second letter which informed me that due to my mental health history I would not be allowed to be a teacher at that time.

I think that the second letter affected me much more deeply than I allowed myself to accept. I tried to pretend that I was completely blasé about the decision to reject me from Exeter, but in reality I felt as though the wind had been taken out of my sails. It was a real setback to be thwarted in the pursuit of my dream. It took me a long time to accept the fact that I couldn't start a PGCE after my maths degree. Suddenly my maths degree seemed rather futile; my attitude was 'If I can't teach then what's the point of even finishing the degree?'

The way my bottled-up feelings manifested was as a brief but fairly intense period of hypomania.

On this occasion it was my Director of Studies who took me into hospital and I'm extremely grateful to him for doing so.

One of the maths courses I was studying at the time was called 'Naive and Axiomatic Set Theory.' It was taught by a man called Angus McIntyre, a well-known professor of logic. Angus became a great confidant during my last manic episode in Edinburgh. He listened extremely well to the mathematical thoughts that characterised that particular episode.

One of the limitations of set theory is that certain sets are impossible objects. For example, it is meaningless to talk of the 'Set of all sets'. To get round this problem, one of the things I did in my mind that Easter, was to introduce the notion of setts, to which the normal rules of logic didn't apply. It was then natural for me to start ranting on about badgers, these being the things that live in setts. (In maths, objects and constructs are often referred to as though they are alive, and 'badgers' seemed as good a term as any for the ineffable objects of mathematical curiosity that we were all studying.)

I was writing a lot during the manic episode, investigating language and logic. One of the things I was interested in was the different uses of the word 'so' in mathematical reasoning. I invented my own new set of symbols, with a different symbol for each use of the word 'so'. My writing became increasingly arcane as I became higher and higher. I wasn't sleeping much which didn't help my case.

I had finished Douglas Hofstadter's book 'Gödel, Escher, Bach' earlier that year. This was another influence on my writing. One of the key features of the book is the notion of self-reference. Statements such as 'This sentence is false' are paradoxical and present a challenge to any system of logic. Gödel was a mathematician in the twentieth century. He is most famous for his incompleteness theorem, one consequence of which is that for any set of consistent axioms there are mathematical statements that are true but unprovable. The details are not important here; it is enough to know that the book is an intensely philosophical adventure into pattern in mathematics, music and life in general.

Partly inspired by 'Gödel, Escher, Bach', I wrote a piece that I called 'Meta'. The first part of 'Meta' was a short essay with the title 'Similarity, Identity and Sameness'. I then wrote a futuristic account of a team game that was watched by billions of beings around the universe. Two teams would pit themselves against each other and basically have a philosophical debate in front of the live audience. As the 'game' was progressing, the intergalactic media sources were busy chronicling the debate (i.e. the 'game'.) It turned out that the so-called 'transcript' of the game was the original essay on similarity and sameness. The final section of 'Meta' was a scene in an oak-panelled room with two of the editors of the intergalactic media discussing the games that were going on around the universe, rather like sports commentators today.

The self-reference cropped up in one of the sections where I used a symbol that I designed when I was in India and defined it as meaning 'That which the author is trying to communicate'. One of my purposes in writing 'Meta' was to encourage the readers to question what we mean by personal identity and to help them recognise how arbitrary a notion it really is.

At first glance there is no particular reason why writing 'Meta' should have been linked with my going high that Easter; it is only the fact that I didn't sleep much when I was writing it that meant that it contributed to my going into hospital.

That Easter the Jesus theme returned to my thinking. I remember I was wrestling with the logical challenge of trying to explain the fact that objects exist and we exist and we are able to name objects. (Although this seems an obvious enough notion, it is not possible to prove that objects exist, but that certainly didn't stop me from trying!)

I built up my own system of reasoning, inventing words as I went along. I will not recreate all of my reasoning here but I will say that I began with the seemingly cryptic statement 'A unit isi a node'. The word 'isi' in the middle of this sentence is intended as an 'is' that can be read in either direction. In other words the sentence 'A unit isi a node' is equivalent to the two sentences 'A unit is a node' and 'A node is a unit'. From this humble beginning, by introducing different types of 'so' as I progressed, I built up the idea of certain units (or equivalently nodes) being labels and almost managed to get to the idea of particular units being able to assign labels to other units, thus describing the process of naming objects. I used the word 'joiner' to mean 'a unit that assigns a label to another unit.' The word 'joiner' got me thinking of carpentry and from there I went on to write something about Jesus. I felt a very definite sense of coming full circle as I tied all these ideas together and linked them with 'The real world.' I don't remember all the details of my thought processes but I do remember telling Angus (albeit in a subtle and roundabout way) about my thoughts on Jesus. It seemed important at the time that it was Easter 2001. To give you some idea of what state I was in, I was talking to Angus in his office, using chalk and blackboard to put my ideas across, and found myself attempting to communicate ideas by 'writing' with the chalk in the air when two dimensions felt too limiting for the enormity of the thoughts I was attempting to convey!

During that period I stopped caring about lectures and missed a few. In others I simply sat at the back and observed, making no effort to take notes. I started making lots of copies of my writing to hand out to staff and students. Eventually my activities came to the attention of my Director of Studies, who, knowing about my manic episodes in the past, decided that I needed to go into hospital again.

It took another few days to arrange a meeting with Professor Blackwood, by which time I was so high that I had the feeling that I had almost entirely severed my connection to the physical world. What I mean by this is that my body began to feel extremely light and I seemed to be able to move almost without any effort at all.

So I went into hospital again. Lots of my friends came to see me, including Mary, who handled it all very well.

I didn't stay in hospital for more than about a week, much to the surprise of my Director of Studies who though I would need a long stay in hospital. During my week in hospital I was allowed to go to lectures during the day so I didn't miss too much.

On the day my Director of Studies took me into hospital he first took me to his house for lunch. I clearly remember the conversation we had.

I was extremely aware of every nuance of body language, eye contact and verbal utterances. It felt as though I was almost able to see time. As the conversation progressed and we established common points of reference I had the feeling that ideas were literally crystallising to create physical reality. Every moment was full and exceedingly clear. I was probably more conscious of the moment than at any other time in my life. It was a very memorable meal.

After my visit into hospital I managed to stay out for quite a long time - over a year in fact.

I finished my maths degree and graduated in July 2001. The only slight hiccough came when I was doing my final revision for my exams. I did a lot of work with a friend who was also studying maths. Mark and I got on well and it was a very productive revision partnership.

Mark had a large home entertainment system and we would watch a bit of lunchtime news or a DVD as a break from our day of revision. I was still a little high from my Easter episode and as Mark and I were revising together for our finals I found myself attempting to use the conversational styles of the news presenters. I would ask searching questions and use changes of tone of voice to put across nuances of meaning. It came across as distinctly unKim-like and Mark was a bit worried. However that passed and I succeeded in getting through my exams and obtaining the first class honours degree I deserved. Having been rejected by Exeter for the PGCE course, I no longer had a clear idea of where I was heading after my maths degree. It was partly this uncertainty and the feeling that my maths degree was a waste of time if I couldn't be a teacher that drove me into hospital at Easter of my final year.

I received an email some time around May about a new master's course that was being run jointly by the universities of St Andrews and Dundee. It was an MRes (Masters by research) in Environmental Biology, Conversion for Mathematicians, Physicists and Molecular Biologists. It was funded by the Natural Environment Research Council (NERC) in an attempt to entice people with strong mathematical ability into environmental biology. It sounded like an interesting course, and, since I was in a quandary about where to go next, I decided to apply.

St Andrews: New Place, Same Old Mania

Mary accompanied me to St. Andrews on the day of my interview. We had a walk together along the coast and wandered through the town. I liked the town and so, when I was offered a place on the course, I accepted.

During my year in St. Andrews I went high twice - once at Easter and once during the summer, just before I finished the course. I ended up in hospital briefly on each occasion. Having said this, I was in an elevated state for most of that year.

It began in a peculiar way.

I graduated from Edinburgh in July 2001. That summer I had a job working as the activity organiser for a language school in the city centre. It was a job that involved taking groups of foreign teenagers on trips; most days the students had English lessons in the mornings and activities were laid on for them in the afternoons. It gave me an excuse to do all the fun touristy things around Edinburgh before waving goodbye to the city that had been my home for the last seven years.

Although I went a little bit high during the festival, when I was trying to organise evening activities for the adults at the language school as well as doing my work with the juniors, on the whole it was a very relaxed and enjoyable time for me.

When September came, Mary and I decided to spend a couple of weeks living with her parents in Dundee before the term started in St Andrews. During our stay we were looked after extremely well. Mary's mum was a fabulous cook and seemed to enjoy cooking for us. We went for plenty of walks and it felt as though we were on holiday.

As further evidence of my tendency to do extreme and inappropriate things, I will briefly mention a holiday Mary and I had in September 2001.

Over the summer there had been a large party of Italian students at the language school. There were a couple of adults with the group and I got to know them well, what with plenty of coach trips and arranging activities for the students. One woman lived near Florence and she invited me and Mary to her house in September. Mary and I had booked a cheap flight from Stansted to Venice Treviso; the plan was to have a day or two in Venice at either end of the holiday and take the train from Venice to Florence. Since the flight left very early in the morning we spent a bit of time at Gemma's flat in London before leaving for Italy. I spent two or three days with Gemma and then Mary joined us on the day before we flew out. One of the books Gemma had lying on her coffee table was a diet book called 'The Zone Diet'. It was a diet geared towards optimising mind and body (the title refers to occasions when sportsmen are functioning at their peak and effortlessly accessing 'The Zone'.) I was convinced by the arguments put forward and decided to implement the ideas immediately. Unfortunately, going on holiday to Italy was hardly the most intelligent time to embark on a low carbohydrate diet that involved eating nutrients in carefully calculated ratios. Pasta and pizza were out and I ended up eating mainly salads. It's ironic that I love Italian cuisine but on my first visit to Italy I bound myself by rules that precluded my enjoying the food to the full. In spite of my extremism, Mary and I had a splendid holiday. We wandered round Venice, had a stop in Bologna on the way down to Florence and enjoyed the sights of Tuscany before heading back up north for our return flight. We were due to fly home on September 12th, the day after the Twin Towers were destroyed.

We were meandering through the streets of Venice when we saw people clustering around television shops looking agog at the news. We didn't understand what had happened until we got back to our guesthouse in the evening and the owner told us about the horror in America. We switched on the television in our room. From the CNN headlines that scrolled across the screen from time to time we picked up a basic picture of what had happened. One of our immediate concerns was whether we would be able to fly home the following day.

As it happened our fears were unfounded - the idea that a terrorist attack in America would immediately stop all flights all over the world turned out to be a naive interpretation. Our flight was not affected and after arriving back in Britain we travelled up to Dundee to Mary's parents' house.

I spent the next 7-10 days trying to piece together an understanding of the import of the destruction of the World Trade Center. I felt I had a lot of catching up to do. I had never really followed current affairs and had a very limited understanding of political events on a global scale. During that period I watched more television than I ever had before, and read newspapers for hours on end. I realised that events of that September were so enormous that to remain ignorant of the wider world was no longer an option. One of the things I started that September was a fictional 'History of the 21st Century'. In my naive and innocent way I attempted to map out how the world could choose to respond to the September 11th attack over the subsequent century. I wrote about seven pages before feeling that without a stronger understanding of how the world had got to that point it was rather meaningless for me to pontificate about the future.

About a fortnight after September 11th Mary and I went to St Andrews to look for a place to live for the following year. I was convinced that we would be able to find a place in one day. Mary's parents and Mary herself were certain that it would not be so easy. We only looked at two or three flats before finding a splendid place to live right opposite the university library in the centre of town. It was a spacious first floor flat in a modern block of four. We had two bedrooms, one of which became my study, and a huge dining room/living area. There was a little shared garden at the back with a bird table. We had a resident squirrel that we later named Syracuse.

Having lived in Edinburgh for seven years and having deliberately restricted my travelling, I was not particularly used to moving around. It is debatable whether I ever felt settled in St Andrews. I think I missed the activity of the capital and therefore failed to fully appreciate what St Andrews had to offer. At the time I was very much addicted to books and I missed having easy access to big bookshops. Temperamentally it was a chaotic and troubled year but it was very enjoyable at the same time.

One reason my year in St Andrews was a challenging time was that knowing I would only be there for a year I felt an insane desire to cram in as much studenty activity as possible. (The reason I could only see myself living there for a year was that I knew that for Mary St Andrews was only ever a stopgap - she ideally wanted to move to Germany and I had promised that she could decide where we went next since I had 'dragged her along' to St Andrews.) I joined the role-playing society, the university windband and the university choir. The latter took up all of my Sundays, with a service in the morning and a rehearsal in the afternoon. Sometimes we had extra rehearsals on Saturdays - it took up a lot of time, time that I could have better used by spending it with Mary.

Mary had an excellent sense of humour, which was probably one of the reasons she was able to put up with my eccentricities for 16 months. There was a bookcase in the big room. My first attempt at ordering our books was disastrously egocentric; I essentially filled the living room bookcase with my books, leaving only cupboard space in the study bedroom for Mary's books. Although she was unperturbed at having none of her books in the public area, it was an unhealthy and domineering action on my part. Later in the year I had the sense to remove some of my books from that bookcase and to allow Mary some shelf space in the living room. Mary was highly amused when I finished the initial distribution of books and proudly showed her my 'well-ordered collection of reference books'. What a peculiar state I was in!

The last section of the MRes course I was on consisted of an 11-week research project on a topic of our choosing. I had the good fortune to work with Professor John Raven. He became an inspiring mentor who I will always look back on extremely fondly.

I started thinking about what I might like to do for my research project quite early on in the course. I think it was in September - right at the start of the one year masters programme when I had a conversation with one of the other people on the course about some of my ideas for potential projects. He told me later that he was amazed at my organisation; it seemed extraordinary to him that I was thinking so far ahead.

In reality, the fact that my thoughts were already on the project simply indicated that I was spending so much time and energy thinking about things that were way in the future that it was questionable whether I was living in the present at all. However, one consequence of thinking about my project so far in advance was that I ended up doing fascinating research that led very naturally into a PhD.

Before I describe my slightly zany research project, I feel it is worth mentioning my first meeting with Professor Raven.

The first week of the MRes was an induction week. The course was being run jointly by the universities of St Andrews and Dundee. During that first week the 16 people on the course were shown round various places in the two universities, or places that had contact with the university biology departments. I first met John Raven at the Scottish Crop Research Institute. He was our guide for the day and showed us various laboratories and pieces of expensive-looking machinery at the institute. When I met him, Professor Raven was wearing a black skirt, a pair of walking boots and a shirt and tie. His visage reminded me of the pictures of Charles Darwin that grace our £10 notes; he had a wild, flowing beard, a big, bald head and deep-set, kind and piercing eyes that looked out on the world with humour and amusement.

During the tour I was the only person who asked any questions. In the wine reception at the end of the tour I started a conversation with the professor. I found myself magnetically drawn to his dark gaze. We looked each other dead in the eye and he thanked me for asking questions. 'It keeps us on our toes', he said. Just as we were leaving he caught my eye again and, seemingly out of the blue, he told me an anecdote that I remember very clearly.

'I was coming through airport security recently,' he began, enigmatically. 'Just as I was going through I was asked whether I had anything sharp about my person.' He grinned as he reminisced about his experiences. '"Only my intellect", I told them', he said with a wink.

It was a brief encounter, but I was captivated. The man instantly struck me as a gloriously eccentric and genuinely crazy wizard-type. He reminded me of a man who owned a games shop near my parents' house. He too had an amazing straggly beard and an extremely engaging manner. When it came to choosing my project, I soon realised that few people were prepared to supervise the wacky project I first suggested. I had a hunch that Professor John Raven was broad-minded enough to let me choose my own way and I was right.

One of my first firm ideas about what to research stemmed from a visit that my Tasmanian friend paid me in St Andrews. We went for a walk round the grounds of the ruined cathedral. We came upon a well covered with a strong steel mesh. Cameron bent down and peered into the darkness. He started making clicking noises, as though, like the dolphins we'd been discussing, he was attempting to use echolocation to establish the depth of the hole. I teased him about it, saying something like 'Given that the most recent common ancestor of humans and dolphins lived er... a long time ago, I think you might have forgotten how to use echolocation.' (Never mind the erroneousness of the argument, the key thing is that I didn't know how long ago the most recent common ancestor of humans and dolphins lived, and I suddenly felt a burning desire to find out. That was the question I initially set out to answer.)

I soon realised that it was an immensely difficult question to tackle and ended up changing my focus, but the craziness of the question brought me into close contact with John Raven and I had a wonderful summer working with him.

In the end the project I settled on was about how the shapes of dolphins and whales related to the evolutionary relationships between the animals. I used pictures of dolphins and whales for the shapes and an encyclopaedia of mammals to work out the evolutionary history. It was an interesting piece of work but because my supervisor was a biologist rather than a mathematician, the project left me with numerous mathematical questions; questions that have now been answered through studying for a PhD in statistical shape analysis.

Just before we all embarked on our projects, we each had to give a presentation to the other people on the course about our initial ideas for projects. I remember one of my slides very clearly. It showed a sort of family tree of about ten species. At the top I had a dolphin on one side and a human on the other. As you moved down the tree, the species became less and less closely related. I had numbers by some of the branch points to indicate how long ago (in millions of years) the most recent common ancestor of a particular pair of species lived. At the bottom of the tree, where the branch on the dolphin side met the branch on the human side was a big question mark - the enigmatic and murky region of interest. As a picture to represent humans I found a photo of Meg Ryan on the internet. She was far more attractive than the usual naked male who is chosen to respresent our species in biology textbooks.

When I was talking to someone else on the course about the presentations, she said that it was the first presentation she had seen me give in which seemed genuinely interested and passionate about the subject. I felt more motivated about my project than I had about some of the other aspects of the course. It was a great feeling to be engaged in my own research.

At Easter I went on tour with the St. Andrews university choir to Frankfurt. I don't know exactly why I went high during the tour, but somehow it was all too much for me.

In the hotel in Frankfurt, I didn't feel like sleeping on the second night we were there so I wandered around in the middle of the night in the area surrounding the hotel. I met some young Germans in a park and chatted to them for a while. The following morning I woke up early, before the rest of the choir. I was in the habit of writing three pages longhand every morning. As I was writing on the morning after my night out, I started thinking about the idea of visiting my birthplace in Zambia. Without really thinking about the consequences, I decided to set off for Zambia there and then. I left my diary open on the day of my birthday and wrote the choir a short note about my decision. I took my passport from my room and left the hotel at about 7.30am.

Of course I didn't make it to Zambia. In fact I only got as far as Frankfurt airport before deciding to return to the hotel. On the way to the airport I crossed a bridge over a river. I threw my shoes and wallet into the water, thus repeating a common feature of many of my manic episodes.

After spending some time at the airport and realising that nobody was about to offer me a plane ticket to Lusaka I headed back to the hotel. I was still wearing a brand new anorak that Mary had bought for me. The day was growing hotter and somewhere on the way back to the hotel I simply discarded my anorak, together with my passport that was in the pocket. For some reason shedding material possessions has been a recurrent theme of my manic episodes. It did feel amazing to be completely unencumbered - no shoes, no money, no passport, no anorak.

Mary and my parents had been informed of my absence and were rather worried. Mary had cancelled my cheque book on the advice of my mother to ensure there was no way I could buy myself a plane ticket to Zambia.

One question I was asked after my 'elopement' was why I decided to come back to the choir and abandon my plan to go to Zambia. What was going through my mind in Frankfurt airport when I decided to walk back to the hotel rather than heading south?

One feature of my time in St Andrews that I have not yet mentioned was the part I had in Aristophanes' play Lysistrata. The director was a friend from the choir. He knew I could play the piano and asked me to be musical director for the play. In the translation we were using the chorus parts were written in rhyming verse and it was my job to write music for those sections of the play. As well as being the musical director I had a part in the male chorus and a small speaking part. The relevance of Lysistrata to my manic episode in Frankfurt is that the performances were due to take place a few weeks after the Easter holidays. Most of the work had already been done on the play before I went to Frankfurt with the choir. Therefore, somewhere in my subconscious I realised that if I decided to press on to Zambia I would probably prevent the play from taking place. Somehow the sense that I would be letting people down if I carried on with my rash plan trickled through to my consciousness. So part of what brought me limping back to the hotel that night was a sense of responsibility towards my fellow actors. (Of course, hunger and exhaustion probably had a role to play too, but in previous manic episodes I had been able to override these sensations for much longer that I did that time in Frankfurt.)

By the time I reached the city centre on my way back to the hotel I was beginning to lose interest in walking. I still had a few miles to go to get to the hotel. I decided to stop at the bus stop and ask for money for the bus ride to the hotel. (My wallet was sitting at the bottom of a river by that stage so there was no option of using my own money.) I approached a German couple. The man had a silvery beard and they were both well-dressed. I must have looked rather bizarre, with bare feet and a slightly wild look in my eye. I decided to keep things simple, and just said

'Ich brauche Geld' (I need money).

'Jeder braucht Geld', came the stony reply (everyone needs money).

'I'll show you', I thought to myself, determined to show I had no needs, and I turned away and started walking back to the hotel.

After an hour and a half or so I finally reached the hotel. In the words of my dear father, I was jiggered. I'd been walking all day, many of the miles barefoot. Sky-high, I'd been burning energy at a prolific rate, and I'd eaten nothing that day.

The choir were not around when I got back to the hotel. I couldn't get into my room and simply lay down in the corridor outside and desperately tried to get some much-needed rest.

When the other choir members returned to the hotel that evening they were exceptionally glad to see me. They had been out all day, giving a concert in another town and had been very worried. I had left a note for the choir, (which I think was only read by the conductor as things turned out), saying that they were the first to hear about my decision to return to my birthplace. They had already notified my parents, Mary and the St Andrews minister about my disappearance.

I was extremely touched by the care the choir demonstrated towards me that evening. I realised how much I meant to the other choir members. One of the singers had some cheese and biscuits that he offered me as soon as he realised that I had not eaten all day.

The next day, we visited a superb gothic mansion, the highlight of which was a large room with a parquet floor that contained hundreds of cases of dear skulls. Many of the skulls had deformities and our guide explained how each deformity corresponded to a distinct pathology in the deer. To protect the parquet floor, we all had to exchange our shoes for felt slippers. When we were togged up this way the well-polished floor became a decent ice rink. We skated round the room as demurely as possible, admiring the odd-looking hunting trophies.

That evening the choir decided to go out for a meal in a restaurant near the hotel. I had no money, since my wallet was lying at the bottom of a river along with a pair of my shoes. A girl from the choir very kindly bought me dinner.

The remaining concerts of the tour passed without a hitch. It was soon the last night of the tour; time for a party. In this case our celebration consisted of a sort of variety show, with people singing, acting and reading out poetry.

During my day apart from the choir, the other singers had adapted one of the songs we were performing to relate to my elopement. The original words were 'Oh you'll never get your granny on the bus' to the tune of `She'll be coming round the mountain when she comes'. In response to my cryptic note and my bizarre actions, the song became 'Oh you'll never get to Zambia on the bus'. Later in the song the reason for this sentiment was given simply as "Cos Zambia is in Africa'. The choir sang me that song on the last evening of the tour. I felt moved almost to tears by the emotional warmth I experienced as I listened to the choir's new rendition.

When we were due to leave Frankfurt the tour organisers rang the British consulate and were delighted to discover that my passport had been handed in. On our way back to the airport I went with a few other members of the choir to collect my passport. We then caught a taxi to the airport and caught up with the rest of the choir.

The tour was arranged in such a way that we all made our own way to and from Heathrow airport. When I got off the plane on the way home I had no wallet. I had arranged to meet up with an old school friend who lived in London. When I got off the plane I started walking from the airport towards his house in Brixton.

I got side-tracked on the way and discovered a small multi-faith prayer room quite close to Heathrow. I went in for a while. It was basic; just a room really, but I felt a sense of peace as I stood inside. There was a poster on the wall that held my attention for some time. It was a spiral representation of the festivals of twelve different religions. I found myself deeply absorbed by the mandala-like calendar, and stood looking at it for what felt like about half an hour.

As I was walking through the arrivals lounge of Heathrow airport I saw an advert that stopped me in my tracks. It was an advert for the Accor chain of hotels and it featured two very beautiful people - a black woman and a white man. They were both smiling extremely warmly. They were evidently perfectly relaxed and happy in whatever tropical location the photo was taken. I stood and looked at the photo for five or ten minutes, simply absorbing the gloriously positive feelings that emanated from the smiling models.

Eventually I moved on, collected my bag and, being penniless, set out for Brixton on foot. I soon came across a hotel. When I noticed that it was part of the Accor chain I felt a strong desire to go inside and write a letter to the people responsible for the stunning advert I'd seen in the airport. So I walked inside and asked the receptionist for a piece of paper. I then sat in the bar and composed a eulogy to the great advert I'd seen on my way out of Heathrow airport. After finishing the letter I just sat for a while, taking in the opulent surroundings and enjoying the sense of sharing the space with affluent people.

When I left the hotel a Norwegian woman approached me and asked for directions to the airport. I gave her directions and asked her if she was prepared to give me enough money to get to Brixton on a bus. To my delight she handed me a £10 note before heading off to the airport.

So in the end I arrived in Brixton on public transport and I was spared what would have been a very long walk. My friend, an old school friend, was very relieved to see me, having heard from my mother that I was high. He immediately recommended that I have a bath and we then talked for only a little while before I went to bed, very tired and ready for some rest.

The following morning I met up with my father and brother at the Bodyworks exhibition - the fascinating display of plastinised bodies by a German anatomist. I remember having lunch after the exhibition, sitting in a park. I was still in a peculiar mood and my attitude to money was still rather strange. At one point I took a 50 pence coin from my pocket (my friend had given me some money) and started playing with it, focusing very intensely on its heptagonal form. Eventually, deciding it was a worthless piece of metal after all, I dropped it onto the floor with a tinkle. This action surprised my father.

'What are you doing, Kim. Pick it up; don't play with your money.'

'It's just a piece of metal, keep your hair on.'

'Come on, pick it up.'

I sat immobile, goading my father. I refused to pick up the coin, viewing the situation as a sort of test for my poor dad. My brother, who realised I was just playing, had a big smile on his face. I think my father felt rather powerless at that moment. He clearly couldn't compel me to pick up the coin, yet in his eyes it was far more than just a heptagonal piece of metal - it had value, it was currency.

Since I had so little money on me, my father had to buy me a train ticket back to St Andrews. On the last stage of the journey north I had a delightfully surreal conversation with a group of biologists who had just been at a conference.

There were three biologists travelling together; a woman and two men. They were considerably older than me - I would put them in their early fifties. I was sitting opposite the woman and one of the men and the last member of their party was a few tables further down the train. It emerged that the woman had just given a talk about sheep.

'What are you researching?' I asked

'We're looking at the social habits of sheep', the woman began.

'Oh?'

'Yes, we've identified certain sheep who we call 'independent sheep' and others we label 'gregarious sheep'. The gregarious sheep spend most of their time grazing within 10 metres of other sheep while the independent sheep spend most of their time grazing more than 20 metres from other sheep.'

'It sounds interesting - why are you looking at it?'

Unfortunately I cannot remember the answer to this crucial question. Anyway, the next stage of the conversation involved the third member of their party, a wild-looking, white-haired man with a balding head.

'Ho, what's going on here?' he bellowed as he made his way over to our table, probably having heard my loud voice reverberating down the carriage.

'This man's studying environmental biology in St Andrews', the woman introduced me.

'Oh, very interesting, very interesting', rejoined the newcomer.

'Where are you from?' I asked him, detecting a foreign accent in his voice.

'Originally from Denmark but I'm now working in Dundee.'

'And what brought you to Britain?' I asked.

'Ha ha, I see you want my life story, yes', the man said with a smile. 'Let's see, after my PhD in Copenhagen I felt a need for a change. I found a job at the Scottish Crop Research Institute and did that for a couple of years. After that I was hooked on Scotland and have been here most of the time since then. Tell me about your studies.'

'The course I'm on is a new one - we're the guinea pig year. It's a masters by research in environmental biology, conversion for mathematicians, physicists and molecular biologists.'

'Quite a mouthful!' piped up the woman opposite.

'Absolutely', I laughed. 'It's run in conjunction with an MRes in environmental biology that's aimed at biologists.'

'So what was your first degree?' asked the man sitting opposite me.

'I did a maths degree in Edinburgh. Actually I did three years of medicine before changing to maths so I have quite a lot of biological knowledge behind me already.' Here I was showing my usual tendency to give people far more information than they actually ask for as though they couldn't possibly understand me without an understanding of my whole story. I've since come to realise that I was rather burdened by my life history during those times. I no longer feel that I have to tell people everything all at once in order for them to understand me.

'It sounds as though you've had an interesting few years', smiled the Danish professor.

Eventually the conversation came round to maths and statistics. The female biologist opposite me was saying how hard she found the quantitative side of biology. Somehow from there I steered the conversation round to the philosophy of mathematics...

...'So, let's consider the meaning of the equals sign', I remember saying animatedly at one point. I was waving my arms around manically and speaking in a booming voice that could certainly be heard throughout the carriage and probably in the nearest town too. 'What does it mean to say 2+2=4? One of the ways I think about the equals sign is as a sort of ball that links together all sorts of possible ideas, all representing the same thing. For example, on the left hand side we could change 2+2 for 1+1 in brackets plus 1+1 in brackets. Then we'd have 1+1 (here I held up my hands to represent brackets) plus 1+1 (ditto) equals 4. Magic!'

The three biologists looked a little stunned both at the energy and the esoteric nature of my delivery.

'But why do you see it as a ball?' asked the woman. 'Surely a ball is three dimensional.'

'My point exactly!' I exclaimed. 'By allowing each side to vary over the entire set of possible, interpretations of that idea, and so therefore the whole equation becomes three dimensional with an equals sign forming a perfectly spherical nexus in the middle.'

'Hmmm...'

We were in the midst of this hopelessly arcane monologue as the train pulled into Leuchars - the nearest train station to St Andrews. I bid the biologists farewell and left the train to find Mary and her father waiting for me on the platform. Mary had a slightly anxious look on her face when she saw me - I probably looked high, only fuelling her fears that I was not alright.

Liverpool - Are you a sculptor?

My last two visits to hospital happened in quick succession in July 2002. I had planned a holiday at my parents' house. Just before I was due to go home I sang with the university choir in the St Andrews chapel. I learnt there that anyone who graduated from St Andrews could get married in the chapel. On that Saturday I started to plan my wedding to Mary. (We had never seriously talked about marriage so it was strange for me to start thinking about it then.)

I gave my imagination free rein and started thinking about a wedding with magic as a theme. I thought about what it would be like to get married according to a druidic ceremony with lots of the guests dressed in long, white, flowing robes. It was exciting to think that way.

By the end of the service I was quite elated. What ensued was a massive shopping spree. (This is a common feature in mania.) I managed to spend about £1100 that day. About £500 of this was spent on books from a new age shop; books on druidry, reiki, crystals and magic in general. The majority of the remainder was spent in a shop of memorabilia. I bought all manner of useless items, including a range of Harry Potter memorabilia, posters of famous actors, dream-catchers, icons of famous people and crazy jewellery none of which I ever wore.) It was fun to buy lots of things, but Mary was quite rightly worried about me. In the end I agreed for her to take me to the Royal Edinburgh Hospital where I stayed for two nights before going back to my parents' house.

I had some very interesting conversations while I was in the hospital that time. One was about the terrorist attack on the World Trade Towers that had taken place the year before. The view that I was putting forward was that the attack was part of a grand unification process that was taking place on Earth. The ensuing clash between Western and Islamic ideologies was, I felt, a necessary part of the two civilisations coming to know each other better and ultimately to unite in some far-reaching new synthesis. The man I was talking too had studied material sciences at Cambridge many years earlier. At the time he was self-employed as a landscape architect and was experiencing a much more stable period in terms of his mental health than while he was embroiled in the intellectual rigour of academia. (He hadn't been into hospital for a number of years and when I met him in hospital he was visiting another patient.)

After two nights in the Royal Ed., I discharged myself in order that I could catch the train I had booked to go down to visit my parents. In my opinion I didn't really need to be in hospital that time - I wasn't high enough to really merit taking up a bed. But Mary was worried about me and I knew that she would feel better if I were in hospital for a little while. When the psychiatrist interviewed me, she suggested that I just take a higher dose of antipsychotic and stay at a friend's house for a few days. When she saw how anxious Mary was the psychiatrist let me persuade her to admit me to the hospital for a short stay.

Soon after reaching home I went up to Liverpool to see Davina, a friend who had been a flatmate for six months during my time in Edinburgh. We went to the Tate Modern Art Gallery and had a picnic in the park. We had an excellent day together and I stayed over at her flat that evening. I didn't sleep much, (if at all), and I was very high by the morning. I flirted playfully with Davina as we had breakfast. I felt fantastic.

When she dropped me off at the train station the following morning I decided to spend the day around Liverpool. At one point I bumped into a large group of town guides, who informed me that Liverpool was putting in a bid for European City of Culture 2008, and that Tony Blair and the Queen would be visiting the city the following day. In my elevated state I interpreted this to mean that the time had come when I would meet the Prime Minister and the Queen. I wandered round Liverpool thinking about what I would say to Tony Blair and the Queen when I met them. Eventually my lack of sleep the night before caught up with me and I got so tired I decided to just get on a train and go home.

I gave away quite a lot of money to people begging on the streets of Liverpool that day. As usual it felt liberating to give away worldly possessions.

At one point fairly early on in the day I saw a tall statue in a park. It was a statue of four angels looking in different directions. I decided to climb up and have a closer look. The angel that most captivated me was 'Liberty'. As I was clambering around the statue a couple of women walked past and asked me if I was a sculptor. 'Not yet', I replied, as though one day I might be.

I looked round the slavery museum on the docks. It's a large museum, much of which is underground. The air felt very heavy as I wandered round. Instead of casually walking through the museum I set about it as though it were vitally important that I memorise every last detail of the exhibition; no wonder it felt heavy!

I remember two other encounters that day. One was with an elderly Malaysian couple. As I was talking to them I experienced something similar to what I felt when I started my natural sciences degree in Cambridge in 1993. Time seemed to suddenly be broken up into blocks. Instead of the usual smooth sensation of time, it was as though every word and every thought was slicing the universe into brick-like chunks. For some reason it made me think of the film 'The Matrix'. In those moments I felt freer than ever before. All limitations seemed to dissolve as time fragmented into a chunky, three-dimensional grid.

The other encounter I had in Liverpool, just before I went home, was with a young monk. He was trying to persuade me to go to a talk about The Absolute. I responded by trying to demonstrate that The Absolute was right there with us. I did this in a strange way; a way that seemed to take the monk by surprise. I took hold of his lapels and started pulling him in different directions, attempting to wake him up to Life's mystery. I doubt very much whether there was much coherence to my argument; I probably succeeded only in alarming the monk a bit.

When I got on the train to go home that evening I convinced myself that I was doing so because the time had not yet come for Tony Blair and the Queen to meet me. (There was no doubt in my mind that they would meet me one day.)

I returned home with my thoughts reeling. I was thinking about how it might be possible for me to find work in Liverpool and for me to live with Davina (who had not given any indication that she had any desire to live with me). At the time I didn't feel like finishing my masters in St Andrews or going back to be with Mary.

I ended up in hospital soon after returning from Liverpool, but before that I had another amazing set of experiences.

The Final Hospitalisation

My father has a beautiful upright piano. It is always a delight to play on it when I go and visit my parents. One recurrent feature of my manic episodes is that I feel an unlocking in my mind and find it easier to improvise music. Also, my ability to sight-read seems to improve. (I don't think this is just delusion - it feels less of an effort to play when I'm high.)

I decided to work my way through Bach's preludes and fugues. I was midway through one of the early pieces when the phone rang. I answered it. It was Michael - a friend of my parents. He and his wife Liz were in the area and wanted to come and see my parents.

I was still busy playing the piano when they arrived. I was a bit high at this point and absolutely determined to play my way through all 48 pieces in 'The Well-Tempered Clavier' in a single sitting. My parents were sitting talking to Liz and Michael in the kitchen as I continued to play.

One thing about Bach's music is that there are few indications about how loud to play the pieces. I have a tendency to play quite loudly when I am high. So there I was, bashing my way through Bach's preludes and fugues as my parents chatted to their guests in the neighbouring room.

My mother has some problems with her hearing and found the 'music' I was playing a bit overpowering. She came through and asked me to stop. I was so determined to play all the way through the two books in one go, that I simply ignored her and carried on. She asked me again and then forcibly attempted to stop me from playing by lifting my hands off the keyboard. I cried out in anguish, thwarted in my manic endeavour, but quickly realised that it wasn't the right moment for me to continue playing and went through to the kitchen to join in with the conversation with Liz and Michael.

One of the reasons I behaved in such a strange way and so tightly clung to the idea of playing Bach's 'The Well-Tempered Clavier' from start to finish was that I was perceiving the world in a novel and exciting way and playing the piano was a phenomenally stimulating activity for me at the time.

What I was experiencing was a fusion of senses. (It's known in psychology as 'synaesthesia'.) I had the impression that each of my five senses was represented by a metallic sphere in my mind. As I played Bach's centuries-old piano music I could feel the five spheres of my senses rotating round each other inside my head. All my thoughts had been replaced by this three-dimensional structure consisting of five rotating spheres. Playing the piano became a glorious meditative experience. I heard the notes as bell tones with extraordinary clarity.

As I joined in the conversation between my parents and Liz and Michael I felt that my parents' guests were trying to broaden my parents' minds. I had the distinct impression that Liz and Michael were using their worldliness to encourage my parents to think in new ways and to widen their perspective on life. Once I realised what they were doing I joined in with the game, using my knowledge of science to slightly baffle my parents.

For example, at one point the conversation turned to genetic modification of crops. Liz has worked for a long time as a biology teacher, and Michael also has a good understanding of scientific methodology. My parents' view of GM crops is a less well-informed views that that of Liz and Michael (at least that was my conclusion at the time). I had the impression that Liz and Michael were encouraging my parents to think of genetic modification as a natural progression from the processes of agriculture that we have honed over the last few millennia. They were presenting GM crops as an important scientific discovery that deepens our understanding of the world and has its uses. Another topic of conversation was money. Michael is a financial advisor. Liz and Michael are well off, and my conclusion during that conversation was that they have a greater awareness of abundance than my parents.

One of the things I remember from my time in St Andrews is a visit that Gemma (my Cambridge friend) and her partner Giovanni made to see me.

Gemma and Giovanni work as management consultants. They are happy, relaxed, successful people. At the time of their visit I was floundering a little in my relationship with money. I was having trouble with the flow of abundance in my life and money wasn't working particularly well for me. One of the things Gemma did was to take a £10 note from her wallet and put it on the table. She then brought the conversation round to a discussion of the design features of the note itself. This change of emphasis from thinking about the piece of paper as something with value to considering it as a designed object was extremely useful for me and it has left me with a poignant memory.

I tried the same thing with my parents that day. I took a note from my wallet and attempted to pass on the insight that Gemma had given me. I don't suppose I made a very good job of it; I was too high to be very coherent.

Along the same lines I attempted to show that by locking doors in our mind we restrict out experience of life. As we sat talking in the kitchen I suddenly got up and locked the back door. I then came back and said something like 'A piano has 86, you know; music is written in 12'. It was as though I was speaking in cryptic crossword clues. My exasperated father said something like 'What on Earth are you talking about, Kim?'

Interestingly, my brother Mark was the only member of my family who understood what I was driving at. After Liz and Michael had left I decided to go out for a walk barefoot. Mark offered to come with me. As soon as we left the house he said something like 'What an amazing evening. How many planets have you eaten this evening?' What he meant by this distinctly idiosyncratic question was that he recognised that throughout the evening I had done things or said things that shattered perceptual expectations and took the conversation in a new direction. 'None', I replied conversationally, meaning that I was just walking my path and what others thought of my actions was entirely their business.

Mark and I reached the dual carriageway that runs past our village. I decided I was going to go for a longer walk than just round the village and asked Mark if he wanted to join me on a longer jaunt. When he declined I realised that I was in for another solo adventure. I ran off along the footpath by the side of the A38, with Mark's desolate cry of 'Christon!' ringing in my ears.

The road north runs next to a canal. I was barefoot and had no money with me. After walking by the road for a little while I decided to walk next to the canal instead. The water was very appealing and it was not long before I had dived in and was swimming along the canal.

At one moment I was standing chest-deep in the middle of the canal and I could feel the slight current against my body. I felt a tremendous broadening of awareness. I realised that this canal was just one canal in a system of waterways that interconnected with Britain's rivers. These rivers in turn flowed into the seas and oceans that cover the planet, where dolphins, whales and other marine life live. I felt an extraordinary sense of connectedness; the whole world was talking to me as I stood in the middle of the Trent and Mersey canal. Awe-inspiring.

Up ahead I saw a bridge over the canal. Its arch was reflected in the water, giving the impression of a single, unbroken ring. As I stood in the canal thinking about whales I began to wonder what it would be like to be a whale. At that moment I felt that if I allowed myself to sink beneath the surface of the water and let go of all attachment to life I could disappear from the world of men and enter the mysterious world of sea mammals. I lowered myself into the water and submerged my head. Contemplating letting go of life I found my thoughts turning to life in St Andrews and the people I knew. I felt I had more to say to the world; that my mission as a human was nowhere near complete. So I brought my head back up out of the water. The circle formed by the bridge and its reflection stood out like an eye. From where I was, with water in my eyes, it seemed as though the circle was a three-dimensional lens shape. Gazing into that eye gave me a powerful sense of unity and a renewed sense of purpose. I climbed out of the canal and continued my walk north.

Along the bank of the canal there were lots of stinging nettles. Embracing all of creation and living completely without fear, I let my hands drift through the nettles. I didn't interpret their stings as pain. I had become a completely objective processor of information. The sensations in my hands made me feel incredibly alive and invigorated. Inside my head the spheres of my senses continued to swirl round each other. Whenever I gazed inside at this new phenomenon, I could see five shiny metallic spheres rotating in a tight cluster in the centre of my being. And the world was singing to me. Every piece of information was being converted into the bell-like tones that I had heard as I was playing my father's piano.

I reached Barton-under-Needwood, the next village on from my parents' village. I didn't really know where I was going and decided to stop at a house and ask for suggestions.

It was about midnight when I knocked on the door of a very large house close to the canal. I was barefoot and soaked through but I hardly noticed. The door was opened by a tall, middle-aged woman with sharp features and kind eyes. It later emerged that her first impression was that I must be drunk, there being a pub close to her house.

'Hello', I greeted her.

'Err...hello', came the hesitant reply.

I think that after that exchange I simply stood there smiling, aware that this bizarre situation had no obvious conversational starting point.

'Are you drunk?' she eventually asked.

'No', I replied, truthfully.

'Where have you come from?'

'I've come along the canal from Alrewas', I said with a twinkle in my eye. 'I was wondering if you could give me some suggestion as to where I should go next.'

To her credit, she dealt with this remarkably well. I could see various responses fleeting across her consciousness as she considered how to reply.

'That very much depends on where you're heading', she said diplomatically, her aristocratic social training showing through.

'North', I stated emphatically.

That was the clinching factor. That answer intrigued her sufficiently for her to invite me in, give me a towel to sit on, put on a kettle and call her husband down from upstairs.

Her husband was a big man with a ginger beard. It transpired during the course of the conversation that he had studied natural sciences in Edinburgh and worked as an industrial chemist. The woman introduced me to her husband in a witty, warm way. Her mother was visiting and the four of us had a wonderfully surreal and funny conversation in their kitchen. It was decided that the best course of action would be for me to return to my parents' house. Since I had turned up at the house wanting some suggestion about where to go next, this decision was as good as any other and I readily agreed. I gave them my parents' phone number and the woman's husband rang my parents, told them that I was fine if a little wet, and my father came and picked me up.

When I got home I went to bed. As I lay awake waiting for sleep to envelop me I was aware that I was still thinking about the five metallic spheres rotating around each other. I imagined myself sinking deep into the Earth. When I got to the centre of the planet it was as though I had reached some massive communication network between different celestial bodies. I felt myself transported to the centre of the sun and from there to other stars in the universe. It was an amazing feeling to be dancing between stars, travelling at the speed of thought through the universe.

After a while I returned to Earth and was once again fully aware of my surroundings in the bedroom. I didn't feel remotely tired so I decided to get out of bed and go for a walk.

I walked along the canal that runs by my parents' house, this time heading south. On the way home I stopped by the paddock of an old donkey that had been there even when we first arrived in the village more than twenty years previously.

I stood and looked at the donkey. He looked straight back at me. Suddenly I began to hear a voice in my head and it was as though the donkey was speaking to me. I don't remember the details of the 'conversation' I had with the donkey but I remember being invited by the voice in my head to climb over the fence and into the donkey's field. I did so and the donkey showed no sign of being afraid. It led me into its little shed and we stood there together for a while. It seemed rather appropriate for me in a Christ-like state of mind (as I thought) to be standing quietly with a donkey in a shed. At a certain moment I decided to try and sit on the donkey's back. He didn't let me do that and instead ran out of the shelter. I ran out after him and ran with him around the field for a couple of minutes. I then received the message to climb over into the graveyard and to continue my walk.

In the graveyard I felt a sense of connection with all the dead people around me. I felt the presence of lots of souls; souls that were waiting to be resurrected.

I felt like Jesus again at this point. After leaving the graveyard I rang the doorbell of the vicarage to see whether the vicar would recognise me as The Second Coming. It was very early in the morning and nobody answered the door. This is probably just as well - I have no idea what I would have said.

I returned to my house after that and went back to bed before any of my family had even woken up. I don't think I slept much which is part of the reason why the following day I was high enough to attempt to walk to Liverpool barefoot!

I had no money at this time (again!). Later that day, I decided to set off for Liverpool on foot. I soon removed my walking boots and was walking barefoot. I came very close to throwing my walking boots in the river. The thought that prevented me from discarding my boots was the idea of going hillwalking with Davina. So I tied the laces together and slung them over my shoulder.

When I reached the next village my plan changed slightly and I decided to walk to Liverpool in the middle of the road. That certainly attracted a lot of attention; it is not everyday that the inhabitants of Barton-under-Needwood see a man walking barefoot in the middle of the road!

The police were informed that there was a man walking barefoot in the road and they soon caught up with me. A short while alter my parents turned up. I eventually agreed to let my parents take me to the hospital in Burton-on-Trent, where I stayed for a few days.

It was quite a memorable visit to hospital. One of the people who I remember in particular was a patient with schizophrenia. He was deeply wrapped up in all sorts of conspiracy theories about the world, and was very fearful of genuine connection with people. He came across as extremely well-read, and threw lots of literary references into his conversation. The look in his eyes was one of the most startling features of his face. He used his eyes like daggers, (probably unconsciously), attacking everyone with his looks. At one point, in order to break through his shield of defensiveness, I took hold of his arm and spoke gently over the litany of abuse that he hurled at me. After a little while he calmed down and I felt as though I had made some progress in connecting with him. After that he seemed a lot less abusive in his dealings with people.

I was feeling totally uninhibited during that stay in hospital and I lay unabashedly naked on my bed (in my private room). One of the male nurses came in and asked me to get dressed. The reason he gave was that one of the female nurses might come in and it would 'not be appropriate' for her to see me naked.

Another memory of those days in hospital is of an event that took place early one morning (around 6am). I felt a sudden desire to sing but it felt like more than just singing. It was as though the Music of Life Itself was coursing through me and I was vibrating in tune with a universal harmony.

As an aside, let me just mention my father at this point. He recently trained as a cranio-sacral therapist. He had to do some intense study of the anatomy of the cranium for the course. There's a bone in the middle of the skull called the sphenoid that articulates with a large number of bones in the skull. Its rhythms are an important feature of cranio-sacral therapy. I have had numerous conversations with my father about the sphenoid bone.

I mention this because it was in my sphenoid bone that I felt this 'music of life' expressed. As I sang, it was as though every bone in my head was pulsating with a powerful rhythm that originated in my sphenoid. I felt as though I was part of some enormous orchestra that was in the process of waking the world up to its true potential.

As I padded along the carpets of the hotel-like hospital, I felt connected to the whole universe in an exhilarating way. It was as though I was receiving messages through the carpet, the walls and the air itself. The connectedness of quantum physics was suddenly more than just an abstract concept; I was immersed in the sea of life.

I switched on the television. There was some Big Brother-type program showing. I had the feeling that I was interacting directly with the people on the screen, as well as the directors, producers and other people behind the scenes. There was a couple who had met on the reality TV show and clearly felt deep   love for each other. The presenter was clearly not entirely comfortable with them expressing their love for each other on live television and attempted to dismiss their hugs with humour. As I stood and watched, sending forth the idea that it would be healthier to allow the couple to show their warm feelings for each other, the scene changed. Evidently the presenter was advised through his earpiece to stop being so dismissive and the camera cut to a fairly long shot of the couple hugging and kissing. I felt as though I had somehow influenced the television that day! I came out of hospital pretty quickly on that occasion and I haven't been back into hospital since then. At the time of writing it is over three years since I was last in hospital and it very much seems that clinical mania is a thing of the past for me.

Epilogue

I returned to St Andrews to finish off my masters. I returned to an empty flat, Mary having decided she no longer wished to go out with me. She had tolerated my mania for long enough and no longer felt that she could handle it.

I finished my research project about the shapes of dolphins and whales and returned home to my parents' house to take stock of my situation. Now that I was no longer going out with Mary, my plans changed.

A friend of my mother offered me a short-term research post in Birmingham. So between October 2002 and March 2003 I commuted into Birmingham four or five days a week and had plenty of time to think about where I wanted to go next.

In the end I decided to apply for PhDs. I recently completed a PhD in statistical shape analysis at the University of Nottingham. It was a challenging three years and my moods went up and down a bit, but very significantly, I managed to stay out of hospital. It felt like a tremendously important achievement to spend three years studying without being interrupted by frequent visits to hospital. After finishing my PhD I got a job working for the Graduate School of the University of Nottingham and at the time of writing I am still working for the university. It is a job training postgraduate students in generic skills including writing skills, presentation skills and basic statistics. It feels amazing to be part of a successful team. I've been honest with my managers about my mania and shown them an early draft of these memories of mania. I feel I am finally getting close to being able to put my mental illness behind me and build a stable and productive lifestyle.

I am engaged to a wonderful woman who is an endless source of inspiration and love. My life feels balanced and joyful in a way that is quite new for me. It is only from a position of stability such as the one I am currently in that I can genuinely appreciate just how disruptive my mania has been. It has taken me a long time to appreciate that steadiness and balance can be desirable qualities of life, but I certainly realise that now. My fiancée and I have bought a beautiful house together. This was made possible by the job I got after completing my PhD.

My manic experiences constitute a fascinating personal odyssey into the capabilities of the mind and have given me an extremely useful insight into the ways in which our perception of the world creates our reality. It has been a process of self-acceptance and a chance for me to grow spiritually. Since 1995 I have felt that God has been speaking to me in very personal ways. I felt guided and supported even during the times when my actions seemed to make very little sense to the people around me. I would not change my experiences in any way if I were given the chance to lead my life again. I am proud of the insights I have received about life and my own spirit. I love the depth of my encounter with God and I'm pleased that I am now in a position to reflect on my experiences and offer my story to the world for contemplation and discussion.

One question that came to mind as I thought about what to put in this conclusion was 'What is a Messiah?' As I have made clear in my writing, a significant feature of my mania was an attempt on my part to become The Second Coming. For many years I was trying to live my life as though I was a messenger of God and that I had chosen this life in order to be recognised as a catalyst for world harmony. I imagined myself as the linchpin in a divine plan for humanity. At times when I was high I began to feel a sense that my powers were magnifying and that I was coming closer to my goal of bringing about cataclysmic change that would unify humanity and herald the beginning of the New Jerusalem.

Interestingly, a lot of those attitudes are still present in me, but in a modified and more useful form. One of the key ideas I have dropped is the need to be *recognised* as The Second Coming. The notion of worldly glory and fame is antithetical to the sort of compassion that Jesus showed for the world. My ego was very strong - it enabled me to construe the events that took place around me as a world drama with me as the hero to end all heroes. My manic episodes were characterised by a desire to be thought of as special in some way - a chosen leader to guide the world into its heavenly Final Age. It has taken me a long time to accept that I am no more special than anyone else. In fact this is in no way a negative sentiment. We are all special and all of us are capable of great things.

One of the meanings of 'Messiah' is a liberator of a people or the world. Herein lies the reason why I agree with the attitude expressed in the 'Conversations with God' books that we are past the stage where we need Messiahs. In the end, I feel there is nothing we need to be saved from. I view us all as participating in a grand cosmic drama, with each of us playing our part on the eternal stage of soul evolution. Each of us is a store of fantastic wisdom, great compassion and deep love. As we continue to wake each other up to our incredible potential, we are all acting as Messiahs. We are the Light, the Way, and the Truth. We all come to God through our recognition of this truth.

Thank you for choosing to read my story. The process of writing it down has been a healing process for me. Finally I can stand back and consider the story of my manic episodes in its entirety. In describing the process I have come to a deeper understanding of what has brought me here. I feel I have truly begun the process of understanding my purpose in life.

Appendix

In this appendix I include three accounts of other people's experience of my mania. The first is Simon's description of one of my manic episodes at the time of his final philosophy exams. Next is an interview with one of my brothers about his emotional responses to my going high. Finally, my mother has written a section about her reflections on my mania.

Simon's story: Being with Christon

James and I had heard that Kim was high again.

We bumped into him on Middle Meadow Walk. He was with May, and some other friends. His trousers were ripped, his bare feet bloody. He was of course incredibly loud and happy and excited. He sat with us at the side of the walk, but almost shaking with energy, appeared to be using all his self control to keep from leaping up again.

James was talking to him. Somehow I couldn't join it. It is strange to see your friend transformed into something else. And he doesn't care what anyone thinks - he seems very powerful with nothing to hold him back. James was trying to be calm, and calming. And there was actually a note of aggression in Kim's voice as he said

'Why are you always trying to limit me, James?'

It seemed to me that James was the only one of us who could communicate with Kim when he was like this, and even James was losing him. I was actually afraid - I had to relax my hand to make sure it didn't shake.

Kim was talking about what I can most simply describe as 'Mind over Matter'. Everyone believes in 'Mind over Matter' in some way and to some extent. As Kim held that matter doesn't actually exist, he was a believer in the extreme.

Then Kim saw William. You could say that William is at the opposite end of the mad spectrum to Kim - he's several slices short of a cake, whereas Kim is several slices too many. William is timid but friendly, and will tell you proudly that he is 65. He was 65 for the full 5 years I lived in Edinburgh. I'd enjoyed quite a few chats with him, and he'd told me about the expensive work he needed doing on his feet. On this day he was hobbling quite badly. He was the perfect subject for Kim's teaching.

Kim leapt up - we all scurried after him - and without so much as an introduction he put his arm around William and joyously asked him,

'Why are you limping?'

He wasn't interested in the answer.

'You don't need to limp! Come with me!'

Then holding him firmly, Kim walked and then ran with him up Middle Meadow Walk. And I thought, this is what religious leaders are, this is what Jesus was - a man blessed with unlimited energy and self belief. It's easy to believe in someone who believes so profoundly in themselves. But all the way, William limped. When Kim let him go, he was a little shaken and his eyes were watery; maybe from the pain, maybe from the disappointment that it hadn't worked, or maybe because he felt abused.

Then Kim was off - walking across the road, not minding the cars. James later said that he thought Kim used his peripheral vision to very carefully time his crossing, but it was enough to make it clear that we had to get him somewhere where he could be no danger to himself or anyone else. We managed to steer Kim to Greyfriars' Kirkyard.

Kim sat on a big tombstone, while we both sat on the grass. He sat like a king, legs crossed, looking down at us. The wounds on his feet were irrelevant to him. For the first time he turned to me. Didn't I know that life is all an illusion? Didn't I know that I can create my life, whatever I want, moment to moment? I don't need to worry about food or shelter - I just need to believe.

I imagined a world of swirling colours and warmth that I only had to be brave enough to enter. I imagined that Kim was a creation of my own mind, a light leading me away from my petty worries. My worries at this time were my finals. I had studied barely at all in three and a half years and I was involved in a fourteen hour a day, six month push to actually pass my exams. Kim was asking me to throw this effort away. I said,

'I know, I know, and I will face up to creating my own reality, but I'm not ready yet',

And Kim smiled calmly and said,

'That is a very thoughtful answer.'

Why was I so challenged by Kim? There is no doubt that he was powerful - his energy, his self-belief, his intellect - and he was asking me questions that no one but a guru can answer with self-confidence. And then, after tying knots in my head, he suggests a simple solution, to follow him in his mission and 'Create'. And I honestly considered following him. But I needed a sign, or rather a test. Actually, I was looking for something to hold on to, something from the 'real world'. I decided to look at a gravestone. If Kim was the Messiah the gravestone would tell me. If it said 'Here lies John McSmith,' I would carry on preparing for my finals. I looked to my right, in a moment when I knew Kim was talking to James, and the stone said 'When I come again, do not fail to follow me.' I felt my face burn red. I stared at the ground in front of me. I said nothing to Kim.

Soon we left the graveyard to walk to James' flat. I noticed Kim was limping. This was the thing I needed to hold on to. If Kim, with all his self belief and power, had to limp from pain, then how could I leave the restrictions of the physical world and Create? I resolved to carry on with my finals.

And the gravestone? I went back to check the gravestone. It said something slightly different. In my fear I had rewritten what I read.

And some people, who want to believe in miracles, will say that the words on the stone actually changed. Certainly in my head they did, I did create for a second. But still Kim limped, and still William limped, and still when Kim is on the right dose of the right drug, Kim is far more at one with all of us. But in the end, I like this 'real world', and I want to stay in it, and that's not just the easy choice, it's the choice with pain, finals, and for me, meaning.

Sankie's view

My brother Sankie is a couple of years younger than me. He is a great athlete and runs about 50 or 60 miles a week. He, like me, doesn't drink alcohol, and in general is a tremendously healthy person. He has done a lot of independent travelling. As well as teaching English in Indonesia for a year, he has made a couple of big trips to Africa, one for an international work camp in Togo and once to Kenya, Tanzania and Zambia, one aim of which was to visit his birthplace. He is open, generous and very well grounded. His current work as a primary school teacher is broadening his mind further; he talks very intelligently about many topics and is a successful person in many ways.

On a recent family holiday in Wales, I interviewed Sankie about his experiences of my manic episodes. He felt that that would be easier for him emotionally than writing his account himself - less of the negativity would be dredged up in a brief interview than if he spent a number of days thinking about how to voice his ideas. Here is what Sankie said:

'When did you first become aware that something wasn't right?'

'It was in 1995 during my first year of university. You came with Richard to pick me up at the end of term. Although I was always aware that you had lots of energy, you seemed full of self-righteousness. We had lots of conflicts and you were very argumentative. Your eyes looked 'too well' and they moved around a lot. Our telephone conversations were different when you were high.'

'How did it feel to think you had a brother with mania?'

'Firstly, there was never any stigma for me. On a personal emotional level I found it hard to relate to you. Your mind was working so fast. You seemed to turn my world upside down. Your idea that everything was predetermined led to heated discussions. I found it a difficult idea to contend with - it was so different to what I believed. I felt that what I said was being undervalued. Your ideas changed so rapidly. Sometimes you came round to my ideas but I was still churning over the difficult stuff.'

'How would you describe what I went through in the first couple of years?'

'Your experiences were lacking coherence. It was as though you were trying to be something you weren't - trying to be something you hadn't been before. You were embracing lots of ideas - predetermination, minimalism - you gave away a lot of stuff! There was no rhyme or reason to your actions. You gave away things that were really valuable to you (your instruments). You didn't come across as being very in touch with yourself. The boom and bust cycles were very disruptive for the people around you. The people around you felt they couldn't do anything to help you. Clearly you were thinking very fast and you looked incredibly alert.

I remember seeing you in hospital once. You were playing amazing music on the piano with your eyes closed. It was like a 'fit of creativity'. You also did amazing drawings and paintings.'

'What did you go through emotionally during my years of mania?'

'I was upset and hurt. I did a lot of self-questioning about my ideas on life. I wondered whether the ideas you were embracing were any closer to happiness than what I had inside.

I thought a lot about our relationship and how to go about rebuilding it. By 2001 you were somehow more accessible. I was very eager to see you again; I could deal with you perfectly well no matter what state you were in.

I remember an outburst at Christmas 2002 when you and Mark were both living at home and never seemed to write to me independently of Janneke and Richard. I was really angry and flipped out when I came home to see the family.'

'How did you go about rebuilding the relationship?'

'After you left St. Andrews and were living at home with Janneke and Richard I made a point of talking to you on the phone. We exchanged some emails and gradually established independent contact.

I didn't think it was natural for adults to live with their parents. You were establishing a rapport and routine as a foursome and I was not part of those interactions. I felt as though you'd all been moving on without me being a part of it.

Although I'd moved on it felt as though I was left out.'

'What else do you remember about being with me when I was high?'

'You were so sure of your superhuman powers. You desperately wanted to go for a run with me. You set off with me. I deliberately set off on a fast run. You turned back after half a mile claiming you couldn't be bothered (but you were very out of breath.)

There was a preponderance of highly intense philosophical conversation when the family was alone. It was only when friends were round that the family seemed 'normal'. I felt a bit left out and alienated. I didn't feel like reading those sorts of books.

I remember a time when you were driving me and some friends home from somewhere when you were high. You deliberately missed the turning for Alrewas and then derived great pleasure from driving on the wrong side of the road. When I got out of the car I was feeling much shaken. Janneke and Richard decided you weren't responsible enough to drive for a while. You were using it as an activity to 'demonstrate our lack of free will'. You felt that it was predetermined that we had to drive round the neighbouring village.'

'Looking back over the last decade, what's changed for you in terms of my mental illness?'

'I've learnt to deal with you when you're high without it affecting my 'inner rhythm'. I have a bit more distance from you now. I can react and interact with you when you're in a manic phase without taking any of it on board. I've matured and got used to dealing with it.

Last time you weren't argumentative in the same way - you would make a point of listening which made it much more of a conversation.

Somehow during the more recent episodes you've seemed more aware of the fact that you were manic and you've taken steps to control it. Your life has obviously been turned over a number of times. You've managed to self-medicate and you listen when people suggest you need to be in hospital. There was a time in Edinburgh when you were digging a big hole in the garden in an attempt to stop yourself from going high.

I found the book 'An Unquiet Mind' very useful. You've had far fewer manic episodes recently;

you've not been argumentative - you've been open to discussion both in high and non-high phases.'

'What do you think of Janneke's suggestion that my mania is a response to issues surrounding relationships?'

'You seem to get a kick out of falling in love. Your relationships seem to develop very quickly into 'emotional hotbeds'. You often went into hospital at the start of relationships; maybe they helped to trigger your manic episodes.'

'How did my mania affect you?'

'Very profoundly. I found you difficult to relate to when you were high with the rapid cycling of ideas.

The first time you went high I was up quite late with a close friend talking about things. I found it difficult to put you aside from those experiences.

I found it harder to appreciate you the way I had before - memories of our discussions were still kicking around.

It led me to think a lot more. I didn't like seeing you in that state but I didn't know what I could do to not see you in that state.

I found it all very upsetting. You changed so suddenly and I couldn't relate to you in the way I had before.'

'Do you have any last comments?'

'You've matured a lot more and the fact that you can take the distance to write these memories shows that you feel it's a phase you can control and deal with. Previously you acted as though it was beyond your control.'

My Mother's Story

Kim had been admitted to hospital. Sankie, one of Kim's younger brothers, had taken the telephone call from the psychiatric hospital and was feeling bewildered. But for Richard and me things fell into place.

We had spent a few days with Kim in Edinburgh the previous week and had felt uneasy about him, without being able to pinpoint why. Kim had been extremely happy, full of energy, exuberant and loud. This was not totally out of character, but the intensity was unusual. Surely he wasn't *that* excited about showing his parents round Edinburgh! He talked in an uninhibited way to everyone - strangers who got onto the bus, waitresses, anyone. He was expansive with his money towards any beggars or Big Issue sellers and he talked excitedly, and virtually non-stop, about all the books, all weighty tomes, he had been reading in the last few days. In spite of all this, his mood was infectious and we laughed and had a lot of fun. He admitted he had not been able to sleep much the last few nights and we suggested, reasonably, that maybe he was reading too much and should give himself a break. When we left we tried to reassure ourselves - maybe he genuinely was very pleased to see us and he would now calm down when our visit was over!

MEMORIES OF MANIA

If we had known then what we know now about mania, who knows, Kim's story might have been very different.

I spoke to Dr Blackwood, the consultant dealing with Kim and explained I couldn't come straight up to Scotland again because of work commitments. He was very reassuring, telling me to think of it in the same way as a broken leg. Kim would recover and carry on as normal. I asked how long this would take. He replied that it varied but that all being well; he should still be able to take his end of year exams in a few weeks' time. His only concern was that Kim was refusing all medication and that might prolong the episode a bit. Kim thought he was Jesus and had 'grandiose thoughts', but that was pretty normal during a hypomanic episode and we didn't need to be unduly worried about him.

Well, what were we to make of this? Interestingly, there had been two occasions earlier in the year when I had been confronted with manic depression. The first involved a student on an exchange visit abroad who had suddenly started to behave strangely and eventually was found drunk early in the morning with a cache of beer under his bed. It turned out he had manic depression, which for him was marked by alcohol excesses. He had to be accompanied home. The second occasion was when a dear friend, an exuberant, 'larger than life', fun-loving person, took an overdose. He stabilised on lithium and in spite of mood fluctuations has never reached the same depths of despair again. His condition had not been diagnosed earlier. So all the conversations we had around that time, had meant that we were not totally clueless.

Nowadays, we would have rushed to a computer and typed 'mania' into Google. In the event, we were sent some photocopied pages out of a text book on mental health by a relative and were indeed reassured that Kim's condition seemed to be a textbook example of a hypomanic episode. We saw that Kim's behaviour while we in Edinburgh was 'classic' of the early stages and that the condition could usually be easily managed and people did not necessarily have repeat episodes. Eternal optimists!

And then an interesting thing came to light. For the first time, we learned that my father-in-law had also had a manic episode at 21. Spurred on by Kim's hospitalisation, the story came out. He, too, had thought he was Jesus, but he had been locked up naked in a padded cell - this was in 1929. At least we knew Kim would be looked after in a more humane fashion! My mother-in-law apologised to me profusely about having kept this a secret but she had been worried that, had I known about it earlier, I might have changed my mind about marrying their son! Mental health problems in a family were hushed up, as they often still are nowadays, because of the shame attached to this form of illness. Although I had been told that an uncle from Richard's father's side and an aunt from his mother's side had both committed suicide, the full implication of this only began to sink in now. Suddenly, Kim's episode enabled his grandmother to unburden herself of all the family stories, which she had kept secret for decades. We lapped it all up. Tried to make sense of it and decided we would not be secretive about Kim's illness. It was no different to a broken bone, the consultant had told us, and we would have talked freely about a broken bone, so why not about a manic episode! (More about that later).

So Kim was now in hospital. Some of his friends had become concerned about him, (he was by now much 'higher'), and they had taken him to his warden, who had recognised his behaviour for what it was - a manic episode. When I finally spoke to Kim on the phone, I realised he was already desperate to get out. I suggested he started to take the medication, which he was still refusing, so that he would be allowed out sooner and promised to take him out for some fresh air when I came to visit him. One of the first things I was asked to do when I arrived at the hospital was to give a blood sample for their research. I no doubt pointed out that it was Kim's father's side of the family that was more likely to produce the clues! I was strongly advised against taking Kim out for some fresh air, as I had promised, as Kim was likely to run away. I claimed I knew my son and that he would be fine, but I did agree for Kim to be put on section.... so that in the event of him running away, it would be possible to get help to search for him.

As he streaked across North Berwick golf course, faster than I have ever seen anyone run, I realised Dr Blackwood was right. What now? I walked back to the town and reported it to the hospital and the police. A policeman took me out in a car and we scoured the countryside, but no sign of Kim anywhere. I returned to his room, where I had been staying, still half hoping he would turn up any minute. Then I phoned up Richard and suggested he didn't lock the back door that night because I had the feeling Kim might head for home - 300 miles, without any money on him; Richard thought I was crazy. But indeed, the next morning, he found the boots by the back door and Kim soundly asleep in his bed. This was the first sign of the many angels that have looked after Kim over the years. He had bleeding, blistered feet and was exhausted and very hungry, but for the moment he was safe. We asked his GP to come and see him but Kim refused to go back to hospital, so nothing was done.

In the middle of the next night, he disappeared again. I had rather hoped that his blisters would keep him home another day! Many hours later we got a phone call from him from Cambridge. He had had the odd lift but had walked most of the way there, only to find that his friend Gemma had gone away for the weekend. In those days before mobile phones, all our sons had BT Phone Home cards. Kim knew the numbers on his card, so even without his wallet he could always phone us. We were thankful for this over the coming days, as he seemed to automatically phone our number if he was stuck for his next move. He also seemed open to suggestions and I soon learned how to use this to get him home.

It was turning into a situational farce - Kim racing across the country and me trying to catch up. A GP friend of mine agreed to jump in the car with me to try and find Kim in Cambridge. We had no idea if he would still be there by the time we got there, but the chase was quite good fun and we had a good laugh on the way. We had no trouble finding him and because he was starving the first thing we did was to go to a pub to eat. He seemed calm and subdued and the most anxious moment was when we had to let him out of our sight to go to the loo! He sounded rational and seemed to feel a bit silly about all the trouble he had caused and then he slept most of the way home.

What next? I was willing to believe that he had shaken in all off and was fine. Our GP who came to visit him again a few days later agreed he was OK. Kim's friend Gemma came to visit and after a few days it was agreed he could go back to university. He had exams coming up so it made sense to get back as soon as possible. An appointment was made for Kim to see the consultant in Edinburgh the following day and we felt reassured that all was in hand. No sooner had we got back home from Edinburgh than we got a phone call from London. Kim hadn't bothered to unpack his rucksack and as soon as we left, had taken the first train to Euston. Having wandered around a bit, he didn't know what else to do and phoned home. I was dreadfully tired, but two could play this game. He was in a strange, easily influenced state so I said things like 'you are obviously meant to come back here or you wouldn't have phoned', so he now had to catch the train to Birmingham and phone us from there. He had no money, so we advised him to get the ticket clerk to phone us and we would pay by Visa. So far so good. We were too tired at this stage to care and went to sleep. At 2am he phoned from Birmingham. Again, I confirmed that this must be his destiny and gave very clear instructions about what to do next. We would pay the taxi at this end. Again we had no idea if he would come or not. If anyone else had suggested something different he would have gone along with that. But, again thanks to his angels, he arrived in the early hours of the morning, tired and hungry but at least safe.

That night I spent on the landing. He wasn't going to escape again. I decided to keep in my hearing aids so that I could hear any movements. It took a while before I realised that the sounds that made me jump from time to time were those of my own movements, amplified by the hearing aids! By the time Kim woke up the next morning, a psychiatrist was waiting in our front room to assess Kim and much to our amazement Kim agreed to go into hospital and to take medication.

Reading this it may seem that this was a very traumatic time for us all. The reality was much lighter. The situational comedy was not lost on us. Of course there had been tears, frustration and exhaustion, but the overwhelming reaction had been laughter. How could you tell this story with a straight face? Some of it was very funny. We learned a lot in a very short time - about mental health, about our own family and most of all about ourselves - how you cannot take things for granted; how you cannot assume you know how you'd react to a given situation; to deal with the moment and not with what could be or could have been; to trust your intuition and not to fret over things outside your control. Our somewhat light-hearted approach did not suit everyone around us and I did fall out with a friend over it. This friend could not accept that I was not totally broken by the episode and that the last thing I needed was 'looking after'. For others, especially colleagues, the open way we talked about Kim's illness seemed to allow them to confide in us about their own experiences or their partners' mental health problems. Suddenly we were surrounded by mental health anecdotes, every one unique but at the same time alike. We are not alone.

His hospital stay was not an easy time for us. We knew he was safe and we could sleep peacefully at night. No more traipsing round the country. But to see him totally drugged was shocking. We wondered what the chemicals 'pumped' into him (all highly emotive!) could do to him and we decided we must get him out again as soon as possible! (In later years we were more than willing to pump him full of anything that would slow him down.) I accompanied some of his friends on their first visits because they were at first feeling very frightened to go to the hospital on their own.

On one of my visits I was sitting next to Kim, who seemed half asleep on his bed, reading a half page Guardian article. I commented on the article and Kim asked to see it. He took the page, glanced at it, gave it back to me and said 'Yes, that's interesting.' I laughed and said he couldn't have read it so quickly. 'Test me', was Kim's reply. So I picked out small details in the middle of the article and asked very specific questions. I was flabbergasted. He could answer all of them correctly. Whatever the negative sides of his illness, it seemed to have opened up brainpower that was not easily accessible to most of us! I could appreciate the attractiveness of being in a mild manic state. Of course, it was this taste of 'powerfulness' that would continue to seduce Kim in the following years and some original ideas would be generated in the early stages of going 'high'. Unfortunately, more often than not, flirting with 'The Rings of Saturn' (An Unquiet Mind) would end up in hospital and initially these episodes would coincide with times when he experimented with not taking his medication - lithium at this time. Another occasion, some years later, also stands out for me as an amazing insight into the workings of the brain. Kim was in hospital after a particularly bizarre and aggressive episode. His flatmates were very upset, the police had been called in and his friends sounded pretty desperate too. Richard went up to Scotland, but I was unable to travel up, having just come out of hospital myself. So I phoned the ward. Kim was called and started to talk absolute gibberish. I couldn't understand a word of what he was saying. I was by then used to rather strange conversations but this was different. I couldn't recognise any words at all. Somehow, we started to talk in French. The conversation changed into a perfectly normal exchange where he told me about an Italian girl on the ward and which of his friends were there. I knew there had been an experiment in the States where foreign languages had been taught to prisoners, to enable them to talk about feelings using words devoid of emotive context. Clearly something similar was at work here. Talking 'gibberish' in French seemed to be too complicated! What followed was a length period of 'mood watching'. Was he 'high'? Was he 'low'? Was his reaction 'normal'? Did he need more medication? Did he need less medication? Was he safe? And over time we learned to recognise some of the signs that could spell trouble. Not shaving was often a dodgy sign. Lack of straightforward eye contact was another. A flat mood signalled a `low' but loud and excitable was trickier! We were willing to be supportive, but there was a limit. He had to be responsible for himself.

After Kim's first episode, which dragged on from May well into the summer, and having done badly in his resit exams in September, it was clear he would have to do the summer term again the following year. Having lost his job at Boots, we felt he was probably not quite ready to apply for other regular jobs and encouraged his application for voluntary work. We were happy that Kim had met a lovely Polish girl. She came back with Kim to meet us before she went back to Poland. During the months they were together, we always felt they were well matched and we were sad when their relationship ended. I often wonder if things would have been different if I had been at home when Kim, and later Maria, phoned to ask for advice. The abrupt ending was very painful for Maria. She phoned us up to check if Kim was perhaps 'high' and maybe unfortunately, Richard did not have any doubts that he wasn't and told her so. We later learned that the break-up sent her into a deep depression, requiring a long spell in hospital.

There were times when Kim was at home and obviously not stable. As much as possible we encouraged him to manage his own medication, e.g. to take a bit extra when he wasn't sleeping, to keep him out of hospital. But at university he was more easily led astray. I frequently asked his doctors if Kim couldn't have some support in the way of 'talking therapy' or counselling. The reply was constantly that bipolar disorder was a chemical imbalance and such therapies were unnecessary. What about to help him deal with the chaos in his daily life caused by the manic episodes? I am glad that there has been an increasing debate about the use of psychological treatments as an addition to medication in recent years. It is hard to combine the role of parent and counsellor, especially with 300 miles between you and when a considerable financial cost is attached to many of your son's episodes!

There were times of relative peace. We would start to relax our super-sensitivity to the slightest nuance, real or imagined! But then a bad period followed. Kim's brother, Mark, had walked on hot coals - mind over matter. Putting your hands into boiling water, as Kim was to discover, was another matter! It was, however, a method to come down pretty sharply! He took his lithium religiously for a while and missed only the first week of term. By now we had decided that to be totally honest about his condition was not to be recommended. Not everyone could take it and I was concerned that Kim's extreme experiences were becoming for him 'amusing' anecdotes to almost boast about. The problem was always how to deal with the 'reality' of life afterwards. If retelling the incidents as funny stories helped to put them into perspective and made them easier to live with, then that seemed OK. If, however, they were told to somehow 'mpress, then that could be a problem. So I suggested to Kim to start to rewrite some of his stories. The whole village didn't need to know that he had put his hands in boiling water! And later on, when it came to applying for holiday jobs, it didn't seem to be appropriate to be totally truthful about every gap. Yes, of course admit he had had mental health problems, if the question was asked, but volunteering the details was counterproductive. We began to understand why the term 'breakdown' is so frequently used. It is so vague, it could refer to any number of conditions; it is also so common that it doesn't arouse the fear of 'manic depression'. Of course, 'bipolar disorder', which has now replaced 'manic depression', is also less emotive for many people.

At the time when Kim had burned his hands so severely, Richard and I had arranged a special weekend for his elderly parents to celebrate their 40th wedding anniversary. It had been booked well in advance and they were looking forward tremendously to the outing, not having been on holiday for some years. So what were we going to do with Kim who was, in our opinion, not safe to be left alone? We decided to ask his younger brother, who had just returned from a wonderful trip, juggling his way round the Middle East, to look after him. It was not an ideal solution, but we could think of no other. The weekend had repercussions for the family. On the Sunday, I woke up with a frozen shoulder, which gave me so much pain that I couldn't drive. I went to see an osteopath the next day or so, who turned out to be an ex-psychiatric nurse. I told him in brief the family story and said I thought the pain was directly related to this. I had so much pain, that even the lightest touch was agony. He suggested a cold compress, applied frequently and made another appointment for a couple of days later. By this time the pain was much less and I could lift my arm again to some extent. I cancelled the next appointment the following week as all pain had disappeared. For Kim's brother, the 'side effects' of a painful weekend looking after Kim were much worse. We found him rather stressed when we returned from the Lake District. He had decided to postpone his university course by yet another year and wanted to get away from the house as soon as possible. He packed his rucksack and went to Holland, ending up in Amsterdam and that is where his mental health problems started. Unlike Kim, he did dabble in street drugs, mainly smoking pot. With the genes, that we by now knew he had inherited, we could have predicted trouble. Having a second brother succumb to mental illness was close to intolerable for our third son. He had struggled for years with Kim's mood swings, especially the self-centred arrogance of hypomania, when no one was quite sure whether Kim was well or not. And now to find his younger brother, who had been a soul mate for years, dramatically changed by his illness, was devastating. In addition, inevitably, we, his parents, were for a while main carers again, when we had just about given up the parenting role. But this would make another story!

During the 18 months or so when Kim's condition was 'rapid cycling', in and out of hospital several times a year, we found ourselves traipsing up to Edinburgh to reassure his flatmates and to support his friends. Kim, fortunately for him, has a fantastic number of really good friends, who stood by him through all his episodes. They stayed with him in hospital and during one of his more bizarre and aggressive episodes, when the duty staff wanted to put him in solitary confinement; it is thanks to their support that he was kept on the ward. I have been concerned over the years that some of his friends took delight in his volatile mood and thought patterns in the run up to manic episodes, and thereby precipitated rather than helped him avoid going over the top. But a few sleepless nights seemed to be enough to trigger another episode. At one time, to the total bewilderment of new flatmates, who had enjoyed an evening of lively discussion and playing around with wild ideas, they woke up the next morning to find a wild-eyed Kim taking down the front door, having disposed of all his possessions in the night!

The hospital admitted to me during this phase that they had let Kim down. He had been discharged several times with no follow-up support in place. He lived independently in a student flat and most of his friends were also students, busy with their own studies and lives. We lived too far away to help on a day-to-day basis.

The question we were constantly asking ourselves was if there were recognisable triggers that caused Kim to go high. We decided fairly early on that relationships played a large part in most of the episodes. The episodes themselves, of course, also put a great strain on existing relationships, especially as sexual promiscuity seemed to feature as a product. Kim's grandfather, it turned out, had done the same! Much to his wife's dismay, even at 91 he flirted openly with the old lady in the hospital bed next to hers. This convinced her that he had indeed gone 'high' while she was in hospital. She was so put out that she confided of similar incidents whenever he had been 'high' in the past. She even suspected him of having an affair with her sister during one of the episodes.

Another trigger seemed to be academic achievement. He would work at some problem day and night, getting closer to the solution. Then lack of sleep and over-stimulation rolled him straight into another 'high'. We were later to discover that decreased sleep can be both a symptom of mania and a cause.

Dealing with setbacks seemed to be the third trigger. Kim had always excelled at everything he turned his hand to - intellectual work, music, sport. He was not used to disappointments it seemed.

It is not surprising that we felt more and more that he needed at least counselling. It took Kim a long time to accept that going 'high' was counterproductive. It was not a useful response for dealing with negative feelings. It was messing up his life and affecting those around him.

And what did it all mean to us? Were there indicators in his early life that suggested this illness? Initially, we did wonder if his upbringing had contributed to his illness. Obviously, the genes he inherited were very much a factor. But had family life set it off? There were times when he was very exuberant and would enthusiastically buy multiple copies of books for everyone - one example that springs to mind is the book 'Sex and the Brain'. We recently took the last remaining copies to an Oxfam shop! But then his father was known to have sudden passions and a bit of eccentricity was tolerated without much rising of the eyebrow! In his sixth form years, there were times when he seemed lonely and unable to 'connect'. Kim had always been intellectually and musically gifted and we were happy that he had seemed, on the whole, to be fairly well integrated with his peer group. And then, it must be said, that his exuberant times were very infectious and engaging and he was fun to be with. Looking back, it was probably only his six months GAP year in Calcutta that had worried me. Things had not gone as planned and when he came home it sounded as if he had been mainly fed up and depressed. Then at the start of his time at Cambridge University, his prompt decision that this was not the place for him. He then spent money on an old car to enable him to sell encyclopaedias and somehow his talk became more 'grandiose' and reality did not match this. But even if we were slightly concerned, knowing nothing about the family history of bipolar disorder, nor anything about the illness itself, it never occurred to us that these could have been early warning signs. And then, we were in the midst of chaos and were relieved every time the 'old' Kim reappeared after minor and more major episodes of hypomania and mania, which were often followed by a spell of depression. And yet, we could understand the temptation for him to return to the '...glorious moods of dancing all night and into the morning, the gliding through starfields and dancing along the rings of Saturn, the zany manic enthusiasm' (The Unquiet Mind).

Kim has asked us how it felt for us, having mental illness as such a direct part of our lives. I thought whether we have grown closer as a family. There are few families who are not confronted by some form of mental illness, especially if, like us, you have been together for over 30 years. I have worked with the homeless in Birmingham and I am well aware that many people with mental health problems are rejected by their families. I have great sympathy for these families. There were times when we were so disheartened that we wondered whether to just ignore what was going on in Kim's life and leave him to it! Luckily, he wouldn't have allowed this - he came back again and again - usually hairy and unwashed! We were impressed by his resilience - the way he bounced back after each disaster. But for many years there was always a tension and any conversation with Kim would start by assessing his mental state. We were always on alert! We leaned not to be side-tracked by him and to be more authoritarian if the situation required this. There were some incidents that we were very upset about. Clearing his room of his possessions was a 'theme' for a while, but the loss of his musical instruments was very painful. Luckily, loads of 'angels' figure in his stories. A nurse, who remembered him from years ago, saw him walking in the middle of the road with no shoes on and notified the hospital.

They were expecting him when we took him there not long after, having been alerted by the police. He wasn't in for long that time, because there was a shortage of beds. Luckily other angels were around shortly afterwards, when, having had a swim in the canal, he arrived soaking wet at someone's door late at night and he was taken in, given a towel to dry himself and was warmed up by an open fire. We asked ourselves what we would do, if a bedraggled stranger turned up on our doorstep, even if he did have a smile and a funny story to tell. I sincerely hope that if it were to happen today we would open our door wide and welcome them in.

The most shocking moment for Richard was in the first episode, when Kim phoned us from London, when we had just returned home after leaving him in Scotland. The total loss of a sense of reliability and trust was devastating. He also had great difficulty in believing that tablets would be the answer to Kim's mental state. And then in addition, he had to review his childhood experiences of his family, on learning that his father had suffered severe bouts of mania and depression throughout his life. A different light was shed on his whole relationship with his father.

For Richard the revelation of his father's illness came as a shock. He knew his dad had had a 'breakdown' when his grandfather died and had to have time off school from his teaching job from time to time, but he had not been admitted to hospital and, as it turned out, had not taken regular medication. His mother had stoically kept the impact of her husband's illness from their two sons as much as she could. But it was not possible to totally protect her sons from her husband's unpredictable moods and, I suspect, his anger. Joe had spent most of his life trying to keep a handle on his mental state, by immersing himself in religion and, it must be said, that apart from a few notable lapses he succeeded.

If I were asked for a list of thing to do for parents dealing with a son or daughter, who arrives home one day with bright eyes, talking ten to the dozen in an agitated state, with unwashed clothes and unkempt hair, full of exciting revelations and insights into the workings of the universe who can't keep still and seems restless down to their toes, I would suggest the following:

Check if they have been taking drugs
Hide all car keys
Put all bank cards temporarily out of reach
Let them talk, avoiding confrontation. You can say it doesn't make sense to you or that their thoughts are too fast for you to follow.
Stay with them.
Don't assume they will do what they would 'normally' do. A sudden idea can lead to unexpected actions, some of which might put their or someone else's safety at risk
Don't feel honour bound to keep promises. They may not be the 'same' person that you made the promise with
Get medical help

And if it is not the first time, remember that it is an illness. A restless, frayed mood, which can turn to anger, violence or psychosis, can so easily be interpreted as wilful, angry, irrational and tiresome. The behaviour might seem to be deliberate, but it is beyond the person's control. And then, I think of what my father-in-law would say about any uncomfortable situation: 'This too will pass.'

Lightning Source UK Ltd.
Milton Keynes UK
04 February 2010
149529UK00001B/3/P